Ubersleep

Nap-Based Sleep Schedules and the Polyphasic Lifestyle

Using Polyphasic Sleep Schedules to Cut your Sleep Time by Half (or more!) and Do All Kinds of Interesting Things to your Life

The Disclaimers

Please Read These!

1. **This is not (yet) science.**
    There is little real scientific data on Polyphasic Sleep at the time of this writing. What you're reading here is the personal experience and collected research (mostly jotted on napkins) of one of the better-known experimenters with polyphasic schedules (me). I coined the term "Uberman's Sleep Schedule" and have lived on both the Uberman and Everyman schedules for almost a decade (as of the Second Edition). I've also talked with, attempted to advise, and learned from many other people who showed interest in adapting to a polyphasic schedule. While it's all YMMV (Your Mileage May Vary) at this point, this is the best data I'm aware of at this moment. **Please take this as serious advice, which it is, but not as scientifically-validated fact, which it isn't**.

2. **SLEEP DEPRIVATION IS NOT HEALTHY.**
    Just as changing diets often means going through some hunger, changing sleep schedules, especially into a super-efficient schedule, involves some sleep-starvation. In some cases, such as with Uberman, it can be quite extreme for a few days (like fasting, to keep up the food analogy). But even when the sleep dep isn't extreme, it's there, until you adapt fully to the new schedule. *Like hunger, sleep deprivation won't kill you, or even hurt you, as long as it's temporary* and you observe basic safety guidelines (which are discussed in detail in the chapter on Adaptation, and elsewhere). Also like hunger, sleep deprivation is not a healthy state to be in for too long – it can have many detrimental effects over time. As more people become interested in polyphasic sleep, I'm hearing more cases of people being sleep deprived for months or even longer, as they make halfhearted attempts to adapt but keep oversleeping or fudging their schedules, resulting in a long, drawn-out period of low-to-mid-level

sleep deprivation. *The point of polyphasic sleep is to get through the adaptation period as quickly as possible, by making consistent changes to one's sleep schedule and sticking with them in spite of the initial tiredness.* If done correctly, the period of sleep deprivation is short and, I believe, totally safe. **If consistency is lacking, however, this kind of experimentation can have negative consequences**. I strongly urge everyone who may consider polyphasic sleep to think long and hard about whether you have the motivation and discipline to be consistent in spite of being extremely tired at first; and if you discover that you can't seem to keep to your new schedule long enough to adapt—you keep messing up, oversleeping, etc.—then please stop before you damage yourself. Re-establish a regular, normal sleeping schedule asap, and then, after a good "reset", you can try again if you feel it's wise. But please don't use polyphasic sleep as an excuse to sleep randomly, or try to stay awake for long periods and then crash and try it again. This kind of behavior is likely to be very bad for you. Please don't do it... or at the very least, if you do, don't go telling people I gave you the idea!

3. **To the teenagers:**
    Those who are still experiencing high levels of physical and mental growth—typically anyone under 18–20 years of age—should not be messing with depriving their bodies of sleep or food, however temporarily. It's just not worth the risk. Humans don't get a second shot at the growth period in our lives, but we usually have decades and decades after it's done to mess about with things like polyphasic sleep, fasting, weird diets, religions, and other lifestyles that may have uncertain long-term effects. It doesn't take much to throw a serious monkey-wrench into your mental or physical development, and there's no fixing it if you do.

If you're interested in polyphasic sleep now but you aren't old enough to safely attempt it, then I suggest you use the time to research and plan how you'd like it to work when you are old enough—the extra planning will greatly (*greatly*) increase your chances of success, so consider it an opportunity.

...Thank you for reading The Disclaimers. Now, on to the good stuff!

Dedications

Like many projects, this book couldn't have happened without the direct or indirect help of a lot of people. This one measly page at the beginning will have to suffice to thank them all, though I hope they know that I know that it's woefully inadequate. If you should be in here, and I forgot you, I owe you a drink. ☺

For the Princess Psuke Bariah,
without whom none of this would ever have happened (at least not to me); my friend and co-crazy-person, who patiently woke me from my first thousand or so naps, and, just so we're clear, whose idea this whole thing was...

For St. John's College,
home of the most intense curriculum in all of bookwormdom, for being the kind of place where something like this almost had to happen... and for all the tutors there who didn't call the men in white, over this or all the rest of my craziness...

For all the other experimenters,
who collectively have learned more than I ever expected anyone would about polyphasic sleep, and who individually have shown me that I really had no idea what it meant to be hardcore after all; thank you for sharing your experiences with me...

For my daughter,
who tucks me in with a glint of revenge in her eyes...

And for my wonderful family,
good god the stuff you put up with. I love you all!

Extra thanks to:

The maintainers of informational polyphasic web-pages; the many people who've emailed me over the years with their questions and personal experiences; my tolerant bosses; my friends; my professors; my Sifus; and finally thanks to whatever twist of fate gave me that horrible insomnia all those years ago.

Original Cover Art by
Conor Sullivan, who was and remains bafflingly awesome. Thanks for a great job!

Second Edition Cover Art and Typography by
Eric Bailey, whose awesomeness is way too big for one sentence; check it out in all its glory at ericwbailey.com!

Table of Contents

I. What is Polyphasic Sleep?

Introduction

Polyphasic sleep is, in its simplest formulation, sleeping in more than one "phase" or chunk, as opposed to "monophasic" sleep, which is what most people do – sleep in one big chunk at night.

Polyphasic sleep is not new! In fact, it's as old as it gets. Many animals are polyphasic, as are many human beings... at first. Infants are generally polyphasic; they have to be trained to sleep at night, as many a frazzled parent knows. Besides "natural" polyphasers like infants and animals, different forms of polyphasic sleep have been used by groups of people over much of history. The most common case that I'm aware of is the soldier, who, unable to sleep for an extended period while behind enemy lines, is trained to take short naps, either at regular intervals or, if that's not possible, simply whenever he or she can. Sailors and pilots, survivalists, scientists and explorers—anyone working alone over an extended period of time, who can't afford many hours of unbroken unconsciousness—often do the same thing.

Because of this, it's well known already that, by taking short naps often, a person can sleep much less than what we consider "normal" and still function mostly without impairment, and that this can be maintained for a while without doing any damage. But what about over the long haul? What about sleeping polyphasically as a lifestyle? Can it be done – and if so, how? Which schedules work? Does it make you tired all the time, or do bad things to your memory, concentration, or health? And what are the psychological, social, and other effects of living on a polyphasic schedule?

These are questions I've been prodding at for a long time. I first slept on a polyphasic schedule for a little under six months in the year 1999, as an experiment. The results surprised me, so I ended up writing a short piece online about my experience with what my co-conspirator and I dubbed "The Uberman Sleep Schedule".

What I didn't know was that, at the time I wrote that article, there wasn't much other information out there about using polyphasic sleep schedules "in real life" (as opposed to over short durations in extreme situations), and that interest in my success would be very high. In the years since then, many other people have adopted polyphasic schedules, and I have tested out a few others schedules as well. I've been mostly polyphasic now since 2008. I've compiled the information I have on the schedules that work, their effects, the practical side of adapting to them and using them, and lots of tips and tricks for making polyphasic sleeping work, into this book.

This book is meant to be a resource for people who are curious about or would like to try sleeping polyphasically. Please note that I'm not a scientist, so while I'm reasonably certain (via my own and others' anecdotal evidence) that, for instance, there are no negative physical effects resulting from polyphasic sleep, I can't speak with the authority of controlled experimental research. My secondary goal in writing this book is to encourage the people who are equipped to carry out that kind of research to do so. I think polyphasic sleep can be a valuable thing, especially in modern times and for modern people, and I've gotten nothing but good from it. I sincerely hope that others will benefit from the information I've gathered here, and use it as a platform to learn more.

Second Edition Introduction

The Second Edition had to happen for a couple reasons.

One, I have a terrible time leaving my own writing alone, and the First Edition was, quite possibly, the sloppiest thing I've ever written—I was *way* more concerned with getting what I knew compiled into a format that people could have and use than

I was with "making a book"; in many ways the First Edition felt like, and possibly was, less a book than a pasted-together collection of emails and blog posts; the electronic equivalent of typed pages held together by string. That isn't to say it couldn't have been awesome that way—heck, some of the best books ever have been pages-and-string first—but it is to say that, picky as I tend to be about all things verbal, it was really hard to *leave* it that way. I hope everyone enjoys the redesign and format-updates as well as the new content.

Two, a lot has happened and come to light in the polyphasic-related world since 2006. Some of it—like the details of Stampi's research—is stuff that existed before that I just hadn't run into; other things, like the Tesla schedule, are new. For years I just kept notes on these things with the intention of "someday" folding them into this work. I hope that I was able to do so without tangling it up too badly.

And three, I've learned so *much* about polyphasic sleep as a long-term schedule in the years since then. I've stayed on Everyman for months at a time, dropped it for a week, gotten back on it for months, dropped it for a month; I deliberately went monophasic and back; I switched between Everyman3, Everyman4.5 and Everyman6, both slowly and day-by-day. I've traveled, gotten sick, dealt with family emergencies; I've changed my diet and my exercise habits drastically a few times; I've moved houses and from the suburbs to the city and gotten married and divorced—It's been a busy couple years. And it's given me a chance to try being polyphasic in all kinds of circumstances, letting me gain a much finer granularity of insight when it comes to what makes the schedule work and not work, and what's (instrumentally) good and bad about it. And while a blog is nice, it doesn't—for me at least—allow for the same organization and piecing-together of learned knowledge as a longer work does. So I've been really excited to write this, for myself as much as for everyone else.

But of course, at the end of the day it's what this book can do for everyone else that really matters, so I hope that people enjoy the improvements and find the book at least as useful as it was before. I'm working on some follow-up pieces as well, that I hope will provide even more value to those who want to learn about or do polyphasic sleep—I have the beginnings of a speaking-presentation done; and I'm working on what I hope will become an Uberman group-adaptation-and-sleep-study that I plan to conduct, if I can pull it off. I'm hoping to produce a lot more in the way of data, and video, and opportunities to collaborate with and collect information from others... polyphasic sleep is, to be blunt about it, just too cool not to. ☺

Thanks again for reading!

Some Terminology

Some language-conventions have already begun to take hold in the polyphasic world, and I will operate within the community's lingo[1] as far as I can without being confusing to a new reader. Here are some terms that you might see, here and elsewhere, in reference to polyphasic sleep:

Polyphasic: many-phases; refers to sleeping in several smaller chunks ("naps")

Monophasic: one-phase; refers to sleeping in one, usually nighttime, chunk

Equiphasic: any sleep schedule where the "chunks" are of equal length

Non-Equiphasic: any sleep schedule where the chunks are of unequal length (i.e. one sleep of a few hours and several short naps)

Core: in a non-equiphasic schedule, the longer sleeps are called "core naps"

Nap: a shorter sleep-chunk, usually understood to mean less than an hour. The majority of polyphasic naps are 20 minutes long, though some schedules use 30 minutes instead.

---

[1] It's not all "lingo", and some of it is not pure—for instance, the term "polyphasic sleep" as originally coined by Dr. Stampi would not normally include the Everyman Sleep Schedule in its definition. However, the community widely recognizes Everyman as a polyphasic schedule. For simplicity's sake, I've stuck with what the community of polyphasers, and those interested in polyphasic sleep, typically mean by their jargon, rather than textbook definitions (where there are any).

Uberman: refers to a specific, equiphasic, polyphasic schedule. Named by my friend and I when we first undertook polyphasic sleeping. It's a simple Nietzsche reference – we're both philosophy majors[2].

Dymaxion: another equiphasic, polyphasic schedule, coined by the scientist Buckminster Fuller. Aside from my own experiences and those since, Dr. Fuller's Dymaxion experiment is the only documented case of a polyphasic schedule being adopted long-term. (It was a success, by his reporting.)

Everyman: refers to one of several non-equiphasic, polyphasic schedules.

Circadian/Ultradian Rhythms: In sleep-schedule terminology, "circadian" refers to scheduling sleep based on the time of day (i.e. "sleep from midnight to 8am"), while "ultradian" refers to scheduling based on time since last sleep (i.e. sleep every 20 minutes). Many schedules include some of each element, though some are purely one or the other.

Polyphasers/Ubersleepers: people who sleep polyphasically (typically, even if they're not on the Uberman schedule per se; people on Everyman or Dymaxion are still called Ubersleepers.)

Monophasers/Hibernators: people who sleep monophasically. ☺

Adaptation/Adapting or Adjustment/Adjusting: The first 30 days or so of any new polyphasic sleep schedule is the "adjustment period", the time during which the brain/body gets used to the new schedule. Sleep deprivation is normal during this period, and strict adherence to the new schedule is of utmost

---

2   We're also both women, so though Nietzsche's original text (predictably) used the masculine *der Ubermensch*, the Uberman Sleep Schedule is definitely a *das Ubermensch*, a gender-neutral. Occasionally I/we get accused of naming the central polyphasic schedule in a sexist (patriarchal) fashion, and then one of us has to point out that, translated without its *der/das/die*, the word Uberman by itself has no gender. It's not our fault that the English for mensch (person) is man. Also, ümlauts are a pain to type, so we leave them out. Translating to American includes translating the tendency to take shortcuts. ☺

importance. The experience of sleeping polyphasically after the adaptation period is significantly different than it is during adaptation!

History & Known Applications

Besides soldiers and infants and animals generally, there have been lots of people that history speculates were polyphasic sleepers, and a few that we know were. Unfortunately, real data is scarce in most circumstances.

There is a small culture of forest-dwellers known as the "Piraha" who, according to the reports of (unfortunately, it seems just one) scientist, sleep for between 20 minutes and 2 hours at a time. It's possible that, because they are a hunting culture (or for another reason), they've adapted to sleeping polyphasically in order to maximize alert-time, much the way some animals do. (It's also possible, as someone helpfully pointed out, that they were waking up all the time in order to keep an eye on the crazy scientist in their midst.)

Probably the most pervasive historical attribution is to Leonardo Da Vinci. When I first heard about polyphasic sleep, it was attached to Da Vinci's name, and even though there isn't any actual historical evidence that I've been able to find to support the assertion that Da Vinci was polyphasic, he's not such an odd avatar for polyphasic sleep. The man was known for being up at all hours, and for getting an unbelievable amount of work done in an almost ridiculous number of categories. That sounds like a polyphaser to me!

Specifically, the traits Da Vinci had are accurate representations of someone on the schedule we called Uberman. Long before I did my experiment, Dr. Claudio Stampi – pretty much the only person (so far) to do a real scientific study on the "all naps" polyphasic schedule – had called the schedule "Da Vinci sleep" in his book "Why We Nap"[3].

---

3   *Why We Nap*, ed. Claudio Stampi, Birkhäuser Boston, 1990.

Other historical attributions abound, as well, and they include Ben Franklin, Albert Einstein, Thomas Edison and many more people. And though there's no hard evidence of fact that these men were polyphasic sleepers, reading about their lives, it's easy (for someone familiar with polyphasic sleep) to see why they might have gotten labeled as polyphasic, or why someone might have thought they were. And perhaps they really were after all; or perhaps they were just weird sleepers without any specific schedule, or with a schedule they made up all by themselves that doesn't fit any of the types and categories that we've figured out so far. (Many of them were known for inventing things, after all.) These men are all described in various places as being awake often at night, being prone to short naps that they could seemingly take anywhere, and being a bit preternaturally productive. ...Which, I suspect, is how I've been described at times too.

There is one great historical figure that we know for a fact was polyphasic, at least for a few years, and that's Buckminster Fuller, the scientist[4]. Dr. Fuller devised a schedule of 30-minute naps at regular intervals (equiphasic) and called it the Dymaxion schedule (he used the word Dymaxion to name many things which he considered ideal and efficient). He lived on his Dymaxion schedule for two years, during which he kept his usual (astonishing) amount of notes and records. Significantly, Dr. Fuller was seen by at least one physician while living on his Dymaxion schedule, and pronounced "sound as a nut". He also reported feeling more rested and energetic on his Dymaxion schedule than he had in his whole monophasic life, which may sound odd, but I experienced the same thing on the Uberman schedule, as have many others by now[5].

---

4   An absolutely fascinating figure, brilliant and philanthropic, whom I encourage everyone to read up on if they like fascinating people.

5   On the Everyman schedule, which will be discussed in detail later, I simply feel rested, normal, except that I have more time available to me. I tend to refer to the unique energizing effect of Uberman/Dymaxion as "euphoria".

Modern Research

Far less has been done in the realm of modern scientific research of polyphasic sleeping than I and many others would like to see. The latest research as of this writing was conducted by Dr. Claudio Stampi, founder of the Chronobiology Research Institute in Boston, and an avid sailor. Dr. Stampi's nap-research appears to have been motivated by his love of sailing, which led him to notice how lone sailors often successfully trade their monophasic schedules for ones that center around many short naps, and prompted him to study the effects of making that switch. He's written articles on polyphasic sleep in sailors, as well as a book containing some of the foremost research on napping, *Why We Nap*, published in 1992. (Mind you, that means that the newest research we know about was conducted seven years before my first experiment.)

Why We Nap is an interesting, if sometimes grueling, look at the physiology of sleep, and short sleeps specifically, but unfortunately a) it's out of print and expensive, b) it's very scientific, and not an easy read for laypersons, and c) the experiment using "Da Vinci sleep" (an Uberman-like equiphasic schedule) is short and, from the perspective of someone interested in sleeping polyphasically long-term, incomplete. All it proves, from our perspective, is that "adjustment" is possible, by showing that a subject put on the "Da Vinci" schedule experienced a drop in mental performance, but then recovered all of it when the initial adaptation period had passed. This is an important thing to know, for those trying to prove that polyphasic sleep isn't damaging to adjust to, but it leaves a lot of unanswered questions. For instance:

- A subject was found who was willing to try sleeping only in six 30–minute blocks, with no longer sleep period. In the modern parlance, this is usually associated with the Dymaxion schedule; Uberman, properly speaking, is generally accepted to involve 20 minute naps, not 30[6]. This may be a trivial

---

6   Oddly enough, all the data I've gathered from my experiments and others' points to a 20-minute nap being more refreshing than 30 minutes. Most Ubersleepers experiment a bit with the exact duration of the naps, but the general consensus is that less than 15 minutes is too little, and more than 25 is too much. Some people do sleep 30 minutes,

difference, but many people would like to know if the more commonly-used shorter naps work as well or better.

- The subject wasn't really in control of the sleep schedule; he was being told by the researcher how to sleep and when, including being given a day to sleep "at will". Since psychology plays such a major role in being able to wake up and stay awake, one wonders how the experiment would have differed if the subject was, among other possibilities, simply given the outline of the schedule (i.e. "sleep for six 20–minute naps a day") and told to stick to it.

- The experiment was relatively short in duration (a few weeks, which is long for a sleep study, granted), raising the question that's non-scientifically answered by this book: Can polyphasic sleep work as a real-life sleep schedule, in the long term, including normal activities? And what are the long-term effects and side-effects of this type of schedule?

- And, of course, this was an experiment with one subject. It shows that it's possible to adapt, but not why, or what major factors are involved. Knowing what traits make it easier, or harder, to adopt a polyphasic schedule could be very useful to a lot of people!

When I planned my second adaptation in 2006, one of the things I did to prepare was to contact several local sleep clinics and sleep-research-department heads, and offer myself as a guinea pig if anybody wanted to study the adaptation process. I was surprised that no-one did, but again, I hope that that will change. (I and others continue to chase leads in this area today, in the hope that eventually more research will be done.)

Additional research is important, I believe. Because while many people are still discussing how possible and feasible and healthy polyphasic sleep is, there's no doubt that the alternative schedules are relevant today.

---

but they're the minority. I usually sleep 18–20 minutes for a nap; longer than that and I wake more tired.

Where's the Science?

I'm not exactly an expert in this part, but I am a big fan of science as a method and data as a resource for making judgments about things (as opposed to, say, fear or ideology). The scientific method requires several steps.

- The question being asked/problem being solved must be clearly stated

- An hypothesis must be formulated that is disprovable and supportable by evidence

- An experiment must be designed such that the results will provide useful information for answering the question/supporting or disproving the hypothesis

- The experiment must be rigorously conducted, controlling for unrelated/external factors as much as possible, and the resulting data thoroughly documented

- Conclusions drawn from the data must be clearly presented in a statement of results that explains how the experiment was conducted, what flaws it might contain, and what further experiments could go further to support or disprove the hypothesis.

I urge—no, I beg—everyone interested in polyphasic sleep to remember that while information that does not meet these criteria IS information, and can be useful, it is NOT science. Please, please don't be one of those people who claims that something is "proof" or has the weight of scientific experimentation behind it when it does not! There's no shame in using testimonials or anecdotal evidence to make a decision, especially a personal one such as "how should I try sleeping", if that's all the data you've got—but there *is* shame, in my eyes at least, in boastfully claiming that you've got scientific evidence when you don't. That's called "pseudoscience", and it's *icky*. Please don't do it.

There exists lots of good evidence to help people think about polyphasic sleep, to make personal decisions about whether and how to try it, and to help formulate questions, hypotheses and experiments to conduct further research.

However, the research on polyphasic sleep is definitely lacking some important things in order for conclusions of any veracity to be drawn about it:

1. MORE DATA, and more *collected and catalogued data*—we have a lot of blogs right now, and a few group experiments that basically amounted to a bunch more blog-posts at a time, but not nearly enough in the way of collected, collated, and correlated data that can be used by the scientific community. By necessity, this is the biggest overall requirement, but there are important sub-requirements too:

   a. More studies with more participants, to compare different peoples' adaptations & experiences of the schedules in the same circumstances

   b. More repeated studies with the same participant and different schedules

   c. Longer studies looking at sleep-schedules over time, and in different life-circumstances

   d. Better better baseline data on polyphasers before they switch schedules

   e. More detailed information on the diets and activity-levels of polyphasers before & after, since these things are irrevocably tied to sleep

   f. More studies that involve checks to ensure that sleep-times are being correctly reported (blogs are unreliable for this)

   g. More video and detailed personal accounts to help bring polyphasic sleep "out of the closet"

Modern Relevance

The future is a tricky thing. Perhaps the trickiest thing about it is deciding whether we, as people, are (or even ought to be) in control of our destiny. We seem alternately helpless and all-powerful with regard to how we steer the development of ourselves, and our world.

On the one hand, sleep seems to already be under attack in many places, where rapid growth and digital-industrial economies are plowing over anything that gets in the way of maximum short-term efficiency. The physical downtime that people need should be protected from exploitation by a system eager to squeeze every dollar from every laborer... Even I worry that some greedy sonofa___ is going to use polyphasic sleep as an excuse to invent the 20-hour workday.

On the other hand, the 24-hour society, properly envisioned, allows greater freedom for individuals to pursue a wider selection of lifestyles. Reducing the amount of sleep people need, if it can be done safely and with due respect for individual rights, seems like it could be a huge benefit to most busy, modern people. Like me, they could gain time for hobbies and relaxation that they might not otherwise have, and restore the balance that's been lost by dedicating most of everyone's entire waking day to work. I'm sure someone will say that to be so busy that you have to cut into your night's sleep to have any free time is symptomatic of terrible things overall, and shouldn't be encouraged. That's not a stupid argument to make: Sleeping monophasically, it's been shown that people need a certain amount of sleep, and simply not getting it will definitely impact your health and performance. I know tons of adults who do that[7], and I always thought it was stupid. You don't neglect to maintain your car right before you drive the Cannonball Run. Why would you neglect your body when you most need it to function well, because you're really busy?

That's true of not sleeping enough; I totally agree. But what if you could sleep *less*, but still sleep *enough*?

---

7 Kids, including teenagers, are usually smarter. They may want to stay up late, but then they also want to sleep until noon, as any sane person would. ☺

It's a common misconception that polyphasic sleep means being sleep deprived. Sleep deprivation is a phase that must be gotten through in order to adapt to a polyphasic schedule—just like hunger is a phase that must be gotten through in order to adapt to a strict diet. **Being on a polyphasic schedule is not supposed to mean being sleep-deprived**; nor does it, for the people who are successfully adjusted. I'm far from the only person to have said she was less sleep-deprived while on a polyphasic schedule than a monophasic one.

It's already known that polyphasic sleep "works"—that dividing up sleep-periods differently can improve the efficiency of sleep, allowing less overall sleep to provide adequate rest while maintaining (or even improving) performance and health. Sailors and soldiers, as I've mentioned, already use polyphasic schedules frequently when it's inconvenient or impossible to sleep many hours at a time, and they're able to perform well enough to fly planes, steer boats, and engage in combat and reconnaissance activities.

The question being addressed in this book is whether napping can be more than a stop-gap measure; whether it makes a good "default" schedule over the long-term. Can you sleep polyphasically – taking naps throughout the day, and cutting your total sleep time to four or less hours per 24 – and get away with it for many months, or years? And what would such a lifestyle involve?

I'm going on three years of uninterrupted[8] polyphasic sleep as I write this second edition (I'll explain my schedule and history in the next section), and I'm not the only successful long-term adapter, though there certainly aren't a flood of us yet. It's also likely that, even if polyphasic sleeping "catches on", it'll remain a minority undertaking. Still, the longer I continue to enjoy and benefit from my polyphasic lifestyle with no major negative effects, the neater an idea it seems. So let's take a closer look at how it works!

---

8   Uninterrupted except for periods of minor illness, travel or other scheduling shake-ups, which I'll describe in more detail later. The periods of being "off my schedule" have been short, and there have been relatively few of them. Also, even though I'll talk more about it later, I want to point out right up front that every single time I "fell off" my polyphasic schedule, I experienced no "crash"—no long recovery sleep – which would have indicated that the polyphasic sleeping was causing me to build up a sleep debt.

II. Polyphasic Schedules in Detail

Beginning at the Beginning: The Uberman Sleep Schedule

Ah, Uberman. Fond memories, for me.

What is the Uberman Sleep Schedule?

- The original polyphasic schedule: "Equihexiphasic" in technical terms.

- Very similar to what's known about Dr. Fuller's Dymaxion schedule

- 20 minute naps—15 minutes minimum, 25 minutes maximum; 30 minutes is sometimes used but seems to be less effective

- Naps happen every four hours—must be precise (not more than 10–15 minutes variation; preferably little or no variation at first)

- No longer naps or "sleeps"

- Adjustment is very difficult but gets easier after 1 week; takes about 30 days to become fully adjusted

- Mistakes during adjustment set back adaptation's progress noticeably

- Schedule is relatively strict even after adjustment

- Time dilation is often noticeable. This causes some people to need organizational measures to keep track of which day it is.

- Many adherents have reported feelings of euphoria, heightened awareness, extra mental clarity, and other psychological effects

- Physical effects reported (post-adaptation) have included increased energy, weight loss, weight gain, dryness or tiredness of the eyes... most seem to be related to lifestyle while polyphasic, rather than the schedule itself. No purely-Uberman-related physical effects are known to the author

In The Beginning

Let's not mince words – I was one of those crazy experimenter types in college. If there was a physical or psychological boundary in me, I was messing with it, feeling it out, looking for give. ...To an extent, I'm still like that; I just have a little less leeway to get really strange about it now. (I look forward to old age, which I'm told allows one to get away with being openly strange again.)

Of course, experimenting with sleep is hardly a unique undertaking for college students. In my case, I was motivated by more than just curiosity, though – I had a terrible time sleeping, and I was looking for a way out.

I've always needed a lot of sleep—the "8 hours" that we call the adult average is, unsurprisingly, shorthand for "7–9 hours", and I was a nine-hour person. Less than that and I felt like somebody'd used me to clean a restaurant floor. I've also always been a computer geek and thus had neck problems, and virtually any way I slept, if I did it for more than about six hours, would mean waking up in a ball of crackly pain.

Being by myself and away from my hometown for the first time did really funny things to my head – among which was trashing my already-iffy ability to sleep. I had bouts of insomnia that could last a week or more; I had near-constant nightmares, night terrors, sleep-walking episodes, recurring incidents of sleep paralysis and choking and even wrecking my room in the middle of dreaming... fun fun fun. So while, in my experiments, I was partially doing things like playing "How Long Can I Go Without Sleep On Purpose?" because they were interesting, I was also desperately trying to jog my mind/body into behaving itself so that I could rest.

The original Uberman attempt was directly related to all this. It was some weeks after my big no-sleep-at-all experiment (I got just past 82 hours before my safety-buddy put the hammer down and ended that experiment), and I was having the worst and weirdest insomnia bout ever. For almost two weeks, I couldn't sleep more than about 20 minutes at a time. It was not fun, and I was desperate for a way out, but nothing was working—music, melatonin, exercise; I'd tried whatever I could think of short of drugs, and I didn't want to cross the line into medicating myself in order to get restful sleep. My friend, who'd been my safety-buddy during previous experiments and pretty much hung out with me constantly anyway, was the one who suggested trying the sleep schedule she'd read about somewhere that involved only sleeping for 20 minutes at a time anyway, every four hours, around the clock. ("I think Da Vinci did it", was about the extent of the information and prior research we had. We think the article she might have read was a short one published in a 1980's issue of Time magazine, about Buckminster Fuller's Dymaxion experiment.) I would have to go to sleep a lot, we figured, but waking up after 20 minutes would become an advantage, rather than an exhausting detriment.

Adjusting

It sounded like the perfect solution at the time, but looking back, I still think it's amazing that it actually was. My friend even gamely offered to try the schedule with me, both as a "control", scientifically speaking, and so that I wouldn't die of boredom and would have help sticking to it. We both agreed that if it was going to work, it needed to be adhered to with the utmost strictness at first, and that's exactly what we did. Naps happened at precise times, and we called each other immediately upon waking (if we weren't together anyway). To my eternal chagrin, I did not keep a careful log of the transition that we underwent, but what I seem to remember clearly does not contradict what others have experienced in the same situation.

To put it bluntly – we'll get into the adaptation process in more detail in Chapter Four – what we experienced was about four days of mind-blowing sleep deprivation. Well, the first day wasn't so bad, of course. Really the third and fourth days were the worst, and after that, it began to get easier. (But those third and fourth days seemed to last eons!) I really, honestly can say that I've never been through anything like those days of extreme sleep-dep, nor have I done very much in my life that impressed me as much as I was impressed when we managed to get through that period without oversleeping. It really felt like doing the impossible!

And thankfully, it was short: after a week, it wasn't much harder to wake up than getting up early on a normal morning, and after two weeks, it wasn't hard at all. After that point, all traces of tiredness quickly vanished, and we were full of energy and — here's a strange word but it describes us well—vim.

And for several months thereafter, things only got better. We were sleeping a total of two hours every twenty-four, a feat which everyone readily agreed was absolutely insane and impossible, and yet it was undeniably working. On a campus of about five hundred people total, you can't fool everyone into thinking that you're rested all the time when you're not, and you certainly can't fake whether or not you're up all night! We had a lot of amazed observers (as well as a lot of people screaming for us to stop, especially in the beginning—sleep deprivation doesn't make you look so good). For a short while, we also had followers: about fifteen other people, total, attempted to adapt to the schedule. They all failed—but my friend and I did not.

What was it like?

It's hard to describe how epic it was for us when this worked. A normal day[9], as I remember it, consisted of:

---

9   It's hard to think about "days" when you don't sleep at night; our lives felt like one long unwinding day, an effect I discuss in more detail in the "Psychology & Sociology" section.

- an 8:00 AM nap before class;

- classes (or work—we both worked part time) through the morning;

- a nap at noon (which often made eating lunch difficult or impossible, but we learned to compensate);

- classes/work in the afternoon;

- nap at 4:00 PM;

- more classes/work (or theatre, or another of the activities we often volunteered for) in the late-afternoon;

- nap at 8:00 PM;

- more activities or hanging out with friends (and sometimes more classes) in the evening;

- nap at midnight;

- then either more friends-and-parties or quiet time (I used to write or work on computers at night a lot);

- nap at 4:00 AM;

- and then we'd get up and go study together at the all-night Denny's until it was time for our 8:00 AM nap.

That means we were up and moving for 22 hours every day. We worked part-time jobs. We took over 20 credit-hours each of classes. We hung out with people every day; we went to almost every party and event (and roleplaying game, cough nerds cough) that we wanted to. We got good grades (studying 3–4 hours every day will do that), our dorms/apartments were sometimes hilariously clean, we had time for all our hobbies (well, most of them), and we were never tired, except when it was naptime. From our perspective, it felt like you never got a chance to be tired—once you woke up, it was only three hours and forty minutes until it was time to go back to sleep!

And that's why we, philosophy students as we were, chose to call the schedule "the Uberman's Sleep Schedule". It really wasn't because it was so hard to adjust to – it was mostly because of the superhuman ability to get things done that the schedule imparted. We kept saying to each other, "I feel like Superman!"

Anyway, at the end of that year, I left school and got a job, and dropped my nifty sleep schedule due to difficulties working it into the whole 9–5 framework. (It is still true that Uberman just doesn't play nice with regular full-time jobs.) I remember crying the first night I slept all night. (Actually, I slept about three hours; the next night I slept six, and then I was back to eight/nine.)

What that experience gave me, unsurprisingly, was a very positive view of the Uberman sleep schedule. Whenever I talked about it later on, I preached my guts out (and mostly just got looked at funny). But I was soon to learn that it wasn't all peaches and roses, because about six years later, I would land a job that had a little more flexibility, and of course one of the first things on my mind was getting my precious Uberman schedule back[10].

Being A Grownup: The Everyman Schedule

What is the Everyman Sleep Schedule?

- A variation on Uberman that developed in the early 2000's. "Non-equiphasic" in technical terms.

---

10   Actually, I tried to get it back one other time, shortly after my daughter was born, when I was hardly getting any sleep anyway. Needless to say, it didn't work – she wouldn't let me nap, and I was too tired all the time already to be anywhere near able to handle the adjustment. I think I lasted two days. ☺

- Most common version involves one 3-hour "core nap" at night plus three 20-minute naps spaced throughout the day. Some adherents report needing two naps instead, or four.

- Additional variants exist that seem to work: 1.5 hour core + 4 naps, and 4.5 hour core + 2 naps.

- Naps should be relatively evenly spaced, but need not be equidistant—most people find they can stay up a little longer between two of the daytime naps than the others, and it doesn't seem to matter as long as the overall schedule is regular, and distance between naps doesn't exceed about six hours

- Precision is still needed during adaptation (abt. 60 days), but afterwards, naps can be moved as much as one hour in either direction on a daily basis with no apparent negative effects

- Adjustment is not as difficult at first as with Uberman; however, it seems to take 2–3 months to become adjusted compared to Uberman's 30 days; one is less tired, but tired for longer, than with the Uberman adaptation

- Mistakes during adjustment are still deleterious, but not as much as with Uberman. Mistakes *after* adjustment tend to be easier to recover from (some users even sleep in regularly, such as once per week, and still keep to their schedules with little or no tiredness)

- Time-dilation is present but usually minor; most Everyman sleepers can keep track of days without taking extra measures

- Euphoria, heightened awareness and other psychological effects are very mild or absent

- No physical effects reported that do not seem to be obviously caused by lifestyle (i.e. spending extra time in front of the computer) rather than the sleep schedule.

...Ah, right, but what had happened in those six years? Well, first of all, I'd gotten into a line of work that was significantly more demanding than being a gopher for the Student Activities Department; and second of all, I'd had a child. Both of those things had an impact I hadn't expected, and that was to make it nearly impossible to lay down for a nap exactly every four hours (or reliably stay asleep for a whole 20 minutes). In college, my schedule was pretty regular, and my obligations relatively forgiving. If I had to bow out of a theatre rehearsal for a few minutes, or tell work to hang on a sec, it wasn't a big deal; my only major time-related obligations were classes, and those conveniently happened in such a way as to allow a short break every four hours.

Back then, I thought I was napping so regularly because it was easier, and because psychologically it made sticking with my weird schedule a lot simpler. What I came to realize is that getting those naps as on-time as possible is not in any way optional with Uberman. Living by the minute-hand of my watch was part of the price to be paid for sleeping only two hours a day. And it wasn't bad, really; it hardly ever bothered me at all, especially since the naps were so short, so the interruptions were barely noticeable.

After college, though, I had phone calls I couldn't put down, meetings that wouldn't let me bow out or be late, and most importantly, a walking, talking, very *demanding* bundle of joy who certainly couldn't be relied upon to amuse herself safely for twenty minutes. I also, for a while there, had a job that simply would not allow sleep anywhere within a 9 or 10 hour block of time. (Several attempts have been made to develop a polyphasic schedule that doesn't require interrupting a long workday. I'm sorry to report that I don't know of any yet that work. More on the derivation of new types of polyphasic schedule, and polyphasic sleep and work, later on.)

But then, another few years later, I realized that things had changed. My daughter grew old enough to be watched by someone else during my naptime; and my job changed to one with enough managerial power to let me take naps. (All it really took was having enough voice in the company for someone to hear me when I explained that one hour a day (each nap takes about 30 minutes in real-time away from my desk) wasn't more than most smokers (and even non-smokers) took in "breaks", and that if I came in an hour earlier I could make up for it anyway.

Uberman still wouldn't work, though: my job was flexible enough to manage to get naps within roughly the right hour-or-two-long bracket, but no way could I get to any kind of precision in a hectic office environment. (Looking back, I wish I'd known that before I spent three weeks trying to adjust to Uberman in 2006... that was not fun!) However, my failure to get my precious sleeping schedule back had an upside: People had been talking to me online for some time about another possible version of the schedule, one that involved a longer nap at night and should theoretically be more adaptable about moving nap-times around.

I scoffed at first. The reason Uberman worked, I thought, was its perfectly symmetrical and rhythmical nature—taking a "long nap" was just a cop-out and bound to make adjusting impossible. Thankfully, several people insisted that I try it before I condemn it totally. I couldn't think of another option anyway, and I was heartbroken at the thought of being monophasic—possibly forever. So I tried it.

That was in July 2006. As I sit here writing this, I've been living on (what I could not resist calling) the Everyman schedule for six years. I am not tired on a daily basis; or I should say, I experience tiredness during waking periods much less often than I did while I was monophasic, and I have 20 hours of usable waking time on most days[11]. I have had several medical checkups during that time; everything is normal[12].

---

11   It's sometimes (not always) a couple hours less on one of the weekend days, when I'll take a longer core or a longer nap during the day if I'm feeling lazy and have the time to spare. *Please note*, though, I couldn't have done this before I'd been on a strict schedule long enough to adapt fully. The extra sleep won't bother me as long as it doesn't happen more than once—two or more days in a row, though, and sleeping extra will begin to make me tired at night.

12   Naturally, everything from my general appearance of health to my reaction times and mental performance was somewhat negatively impacted during the adjustment period—this is a normal result of sleep deprivation. However, within a few weeks everything was back to normal, and I've been in excellent health since.

Everyman vs. Uberman: A Detailed Comparison

I find that while the majority of people are *interested* in the Uberman Sleep Schedule up front, many more people actually wind up *doing* the Everyman schedule. This isn't hard to understand, since most people have jobs and/or families or other responsibilities that they can't sacrifice to a draconian sleep-schedule, no matter how amazingly cool it is. Everyman is definitely easier, in that it doesn't require as much discipline to attain or sustain. However, if you define "easier" as "effortless to live on", I actually have found Uberman better in that regard.

Early Adjustment

Everyman's adjustment period is gentler but much longer—3–6 weeks for tiredness to fully dissipate, as compared to Uberman's 1–3 weeks. Personally, I find dealing with mild tiredness for that long to be much tougher than dealing with acute-as-heck tiredness for a week or two.

Long-Term Adjustment

Since Uberman is such a huge fundamental change, it has its own inertia; once you wrap your life around it, it tends to want to keep chugging along that way. Everyman, by contrast, is easier to "fall out of the habit of", even after you've been doing it for years. (It's also easy to fall back *into* the habit of, in my experience. It's possible that this is true of polyphasic sleep in general—see the section on "Permanent Adaptation" for more on this.)

"Pure" Polyphasic

Some claim that Everyman is an "inferior" schedule to Uberman—and in some ways, I suppose it is. It doesn't produce the "feeling of being Superman" to have just a few extra hours of time available per day; and it's lacking most of the cool psychological effects of Uberman. It doesn't feel the same to be on Everyman as Uberman. Because of that, it sometimes seems that **Uberman is qualitatively different, in a class all its own**; some people call Uberman "pure" polyphasic, and I don't object to that. **Everyman is a compromise**; it gives a person some extra time while letting them retain some flexibility—at the cost of some efficiency. That said, it has its own benefits, and which schedule is really "better" depends entirely on the person sleeping on it, and his or her lifestyle.

Tiredness

Everyman does not magically eliminate the feeling of tiredness from one's life like Uberman can seem to. As with a monophasic schedule where one must often go to bed before one is ready, and sometimes wake up when one is still tired, on Everyman those things still happen sometimes, depending on how the naps are placed and with how much variation they're executed. On Uberman—with a little luck and a lot of effort—that feeling of "ugh what I have to sleep/wake up *now*?" almost never happens at all. The schedule is just so regular, I think (and so efficient, I propose) that tiredness is simply eliminated.

On Everyman, I am tired significantly less often that I ever was while being monophasic. I sometimes feel energetic and "full of vim" in ways that I think I can attribute to my Everyman schedule, but it's a trickle compared to the feeling of being on Uberman. On Uberman I was *never* tired (after adaptation); for a while there I clean forgot what it was like to be tired. My energy-level was consistently higher than I remember it ever being before or since—some of which can probably be attributed to being 20 years old and surrounded by intellectual stimulation—but that I felt so energetic and never-tired for six straight months, I attribute to the sleeping-schedule. (I wasn't doing anything else during that time that would account for it, especially considering the fact that I was literally sleeping a total of two hours a day.) My partner-in-crime at the time reported basically the same experience that I did: **We bounded out of bed at the end of the naps, ran smoothly in high gear for three hours thirty-five minutes, yawned once or twice and got drowsy immediately before naptime, fell asleep for the nap in less than a minute usually, slept like a rock and then jumped right back to it**. Waking up from a nap on that schedule feels like waking up after a long, restful, unbroken night's sleep; in fact, the sensation of being so completely awake and rested after such a short time tends to really mess with people's heads at first. Because of how rested you are, to your "internal clock" it often feels like eight hours or more have passed[13] . Every person who's ever talked with me about adapting to Uberman has referred to this confusion about time, which after a few days becomes quite pronounced, leading to a lot of head-scratching and compulsive watch-consulting until one gets used to it.

On Everyman, by contrast, waking up from the "core nap" feels like waking up on a relatively easy but normal weekend morning; I feel rested, but there is some inertia. Besides getting sleepy before my scheduled nap-times (which still happens, but I can't set my clock by it like I used to be able to with Uberman), I do occasionally yawn in the morning, or in the couple hours before "bedtime" (my core nap) at night. I don't often gripe about being tired, or wish that I could stop what I was doing and get some sleep; two things that happen constantly when I'm monophasic. But I do kind of dread 4:00 AM on cold mornings!

One thing I think deserves consideration when discussing tiredness, though, is whether the tiredness I and others tend to experience on the Everyman schedule isn't in some way related to the practice of "scooting" naps. Here's my current theory: On Uberman, the effect of scooting a nap is so harsh that you basically can't do it—even after becoming fully adjusted, nap-modification needs to remain minimal. If you're even 10 or 15 minutes late getting to sleep, you feel it; you sleep deeper and yawn when you wake up. If you fudge a nap by 30 minutes, you almost might as well not have taken it; you'll either have trouble getting to sleep, or you'll sleep too deeply and be tired when you wake up, and not really feel back to 100% until you've had another, properly-timed, nap. (Note that a few people have told me that they were able to move a nap on Uberman, though usually it involves moving one particular nap by a set amount that's then adhered to every day. And even that kind of scooting doesn't seem to work for those who've been adapted for less than three or four months.)

On Everyman, however, you can move a nap by 30 minutes without any effect (all else being equal); and with 4.5-hour or longer core-naps, you can move a nap by an hour in either direction, for a total of two hours' "leeway" in getting your naps.

---

13   And also possibly due to neurotransmitters like DMT, which affect the perception of time.

The thing is, though, people tend to be on Everyman in the first place because they need that flexibility, so almost all of us make use of it; whereas people who try Uberman usually (if they've done their reading) expect the strictness of getting the naps on time, and if they succeed at adjusting, it's because their naps were strictly-timed—so they're more likely to keep to their strict schedules. Sleepers adjusting to Everyman almost always find that the adaptation takes longer... maybe this is just the nature of that schedule, but maybe also it's because they're scooting their naps. **Would an Everyman schedule where the naps were placed at perfect intervals and adhered to without any scooting, produce less tiredness than an Everyman schedule as usually practiced?** ...Maybe someday I'll get around to that experiment, too. ☺

Euphoria/Waking Energy

Everyman is completely worth it and I'm very grateful to be able to use it to make my life better—which it does—but, in all seriousness, if I could get my Uberman schedule back, I wouldn't hesitate to. Besides the total lack of tiredness, my normal daily energy-level felt greatly increased, which I interpreted at the time as a kind of euphoria; but now I don't think "euphoria" is the best word for it. I wasn't high, just very awake. I didn't have trouble relaxing, or feel jittery (unless I had coffee, which affected me more than usual when I was on Uberman). I simply felt on the razor's edge of completely-awake most of the time. It was an exceptionally pleasant experience, feeling like that, so then again maybe "euphoria" doesn't completely miss the mark. I would normally be willing to write off this feeling as not related to the sleep schedule itself, simply because it seems so subjective and so subject-able to any number of factors. But the fact is, besides my partner at the time who reported the same feelings, **almost every successful adapter to Uberman that I've ever spoken to has reported the same thing**, even if they claimed not to know that I'd experienced it.

On Everyman, I have, not Uberman-type energy, but still, more energy than I do when I sleep well all night. It's not noticeable all the time, but when I think about it over a period of months or years, there is a definite increase in my energy when I'm polyphasic and sleeping on Everyman. (A big caveat about using that as real data: around the time I took up the Everyman schedule, I also began studying martial arts, and have continued to since. No doubt this may be part of, or even the whole reason for my increased energy. Perhaps having extra time to pursue the things that relax and energize me played into it as well. Also, see the new section "Going Back To Monophasic" for more comparisons between Everyman and monophasic sleep.) Not only do I have more time on Everyman than a "normal" schedule, but my average wakefulness over that period of time is greater than my average wakefulness over the period of time I'm awake when I'm awake all day. That's another point in favor of polyphasic sleep in general, I think—but when it comes to comparing the amount and quality of energy felt during a typical day, Uberman wins hands down.

Attitude

Everyman doesn't affect my attitude much, I think, other than to make me less cranky late in the workday and when I come home from work. I used to always feel so worn out by 5 or 6 in the evening, after twelve or so straight hours awake, and it would make me quite irritable—but on Everyman, I've had a nap at one or so, and I'm getting another one about seven, so at worst I'm a tad weary from the commute.

Uberman, once again, is a whole different story. At the time I did Uberman, I lived on a small campus packed with several hundred complete strangers. To have an entire mini-day-long break every night where I could easily see no-one but myself and/or my BFF was an amazing gift, and I'm sure it helped me a lot. Plus, I'm cursed with insatiable curiosity about everything ever, and in such an interesting environment as a small liberal-arts college, I had no trouble enjoying most of my extra time, so my memory of the time is very positive. My attitude may not have always been positive—for one thing, at that age I had more than a little capital-A Attitude going on. But I felt great, and feeling great is certainly conducive to a better attitude than otherwise.

I think I would characterize Uberman's effect on attitude as *intense*, rather than inherently positive or negative. People's attitudes can be negatively affected by Uberman, I find, when their lifestyles don't provide or allow the right things for them to do with the time they gain from the schedule. I would encourage anyone contemplating that schedule to give extra thought to how they'll spend the time, including what their planned activities do in terms of what percentage of total time spent:

- indoors and out,

- standing and sitting,

- alone and in company,

- in lighted and dark places,

- working and playing,

- etc.

...And just because I'm a fan of human autohacking, I want to mention that **you can also use polyphasic adaptation to create change in your life**, with a little forethought. As an example, when I started the Everyman experiment, I knew that I wanted to spend a greater percentage of my total time writing that I currently did... but I didn't want to spend much more of my total time in front of a computer, at least not without doing something to counteract the possible chiropractic consequences. I realized that I could indeed use some of the extra time for writing, but that with four extra hours a day, there was also room to use some of it for exercise. So I signed up for those Taiji classes I'd been eyeballing for over a year—and which before would have cut into my only available writing-time. This little trick not only saved me some neck-pain, but paying for the classes inadvertently helped keep me writing. (Without which this book wouldn't exist, I should add.) ☺

Uberman and Everyman are, for now, the schedules most used by polyphasic sleepers. There are other polyphasic schedules that deserve attention, either because they seem to work, or because they don't. Let's cover them, and what the "formula" is, if there is one, for creating a polyphasic schedule.

Other Schedules (The "Formula")

I'll confess, I was surprised when people began letting me know that they seemed to have discovered a formula of sorts for developing a polyphasic schedule[14]. Truth be told, I'm hesitant to talk about it, because one of my goals in communicating with the public about polyphasic sleep has been to discourage unsafe behavior; and experimenting with different schedule-types, if you're not already a seasoned polyphaser and moreover, very careful with yourself, is definitely unwise, if not outright unsafe.

So, disclaimer: I urge everyone, if you've never done polyphasic sleep and you're interested in it, start with a known good schedule like Everyman3 or Uberman, and don't experiment further until you're familiar with what polyphasic sleep is like. To do otherwise is to risk messing up your existing sleep schedule, without having a workable one to replace it with. By doing that, you may inadvertently train your brain out of sleeping on any schedule, which may make it difficult or impossible to get restful sleep. This could result in the need for medical care and/or drug treatment to fix things, and you risk hurting yourself in the meantime from being too sleep-deprived. Please don't go there!

However, I'm not the type to outright withhold information (once it's been properly Disclaimed ☺), so here's what I know about the Formula.

- Naps of 20 minutes seem to be generally more efficient than longer or shorter naps;

- "Core naps" or long sleeps that happen in multiples of 90 minutes also seem to be easier to wake from and provide better rest, though 45-minute intervals or multiples of them have also been suggested;

- Tiredness and decreased performance seem to set in once a polyphaser has been awake more than 6 hours, and the longer past that one is awake, the less efficient a nap is at erasing that tiredness completely;

---

14   Which just goes to show, for every crackpot on the Internet, there are at least one and a half closet geniuses. (What the half a genius is there for, I'm not sure, but I bet there's a web-forum for them somewhere.)

- Each 90-minute core sleep seems to take the place of about (not exactly) one and a half 20-minute naps.

Thus, a rough outline of "the formula" for workable schedules would look like this:

Naps	Core
6	0 (Uberman)
4–5	90 min (1.5-hour Everyman)
3–4	3 hr (3-hour or "standard" Everyman)
2	4.5 hr (4.5-hour Everyman)
1	6 hr (biphasic)

A note about that last one: There are several different types of schedule that get called (not inaccurately) "biphasic":

- The first is the Everyman variant in my Formula outline: Six hours' core sleep and one 20-minute nap. This schedule "breaks the rule" of not staying awake longer than 6h at a time, and I've never known anyone to be on it long-term. It does seem to work well as an "emergency substitute" schedule for people on Everyman who are forced to miss naps; I've done this myself and will discuss it in more detail later.

- The second is the "siesta schedule", without a doubt the best-tested and most easy-to-recommend type of polyphasic schedule. The Siesta's nap is much longer than 20 minutes, though—typically at least 45 minutes, up to 2 hours. Siesta sleepers usually sleep 4–7 hours at night, depending on their individual needs. Numerous studies have shown it to be at least as good as, and often better than, monophasic sleep. Whole cultures have done it for centuries, and some continue to. It's widely known that people suffer a dip in energy in the afternoon, and that a nap does wonders for that; there are books on it[15] and on the surprising amount of famous figures who greatly valued a long afternoon nap and less sleep at night. People sometimes argue whether the Siesta is "properly" polyphasic; I don't think it matters, but it is important that this schedule works, if only as a counter to the claims of some people that sleep can't healthily be broken into chunks.

- The third type of "biphasic" I hear about occasionally is one where sleep is split into two equal chunks. The proposed length of each nap is usually three hours. (Two people have mentioned a 4x1.5-hour variant to me as well.) I've never heard of this working at all; people occasionally tell me that they're going to try it, and then I don't hear anything else, which for me is pretty good evidence that it doesn't work, though of course that can't be conclusively decided until at least one person (preferably more) does a well-documented, proper (strict) attempt at adapting to it. Barring more studies, though, I don't recommend this one—or any of the other schedules that don't fit the Formula, for that matter.

The Formula is far from a sure thing, but as the schedules it produces are the ones that so far we know work, I suspect it has some merit. I believe it makes a good guideline for people to help them choose a schedule: Formula schedules are likely to work—maybe not for you, but they give you a place to start thinking from.

There's a big Chart of all the Known Polyphasic Schedules in the Appendices, but the ones you want to know about for sure, and stick with if you're just starting out and want the best chance of successfully adapting, are these, the tried-and-true ones. These have been done by the most people with the highest percentage of success:

---

15   For example, *The Art of Napping*, by Dr. William A. Anthony, ISBN978-0-943914-82-4, which I haven't read all of, but have really enjoyed so far.

Tried & True Polyphasic Schedules

Uberman

Six 20-minute naps per 24 hours, spaced at even intervals

Everyman3

One 3-hour core nap and three or four 20-minute naps, spaced evenly-ish

Everyman4

One 4.5-hour core nap and two or three 20-minute naps, spaced evenly-ish

Even More Schedules

The following are all new polyphasic schedules, developed by experimenters and the growing polyphasic community. They haven't been done by very many people yet and should be considered highly experimental (even moreso than polyphasic sleep as a whole). However, without enough research to say why polyphasic schedules work, it's not possible to say which of these will work and which won't, so it's good to know they're out there. I've always liked the Chinese proverb, "One who says something is impossible should not get in the way of one who is doing it."

The "Tesla" Schedule

Back in 2009, a polyphaser named Sharif alerted me to a schedule he and a friend were trying, which they (very classily) named the "Tesla Schedule". A hybrid of Uberman (20min per 4h) and Dymaxion (30min per 6h), Tesla is envisioned as 20-minute naps *every six hours*.

Yes. Someone figured out a *more restrictive* schedule than Uberman.

Gotta love the Internet. ☺

You can read Sharif's writeup (at least, it's still there as of the writing of the Second Edition) at http://tombstone.tesser.org/tesser/sleep/tesla —and as for other adapters, I've heard whispers of a few, but never any proven reports.

There is a good argument to be made that perhaps Tesla is easier than Dymaxion (Sharif says it was easier to adapt to, anyway) because a 20-minute nap is easier to maintain, and feel rested from, than a 30-minute nap. That's my experience too... but I'm not sure I could do *any* length nap every *six* hours with no other sleep. Obviously more information is needed to make any real determination on Tesla's applicability and practicality; maybe it's only really suitable for people who need less sleep normally.

Circadian Triphasic

This interesting name (coined by an experimenter writing as "Leif") refers to three equally-spaced 1.5 hour core naps. I've spoken to several people who successfully adapted to it, and as a bonus the adjustment process is reported to be relatively easy as well. Getting an hour and a half to sleep during the day seems to be the big challenge with this one.

SPAMAYL

The fun-to-say acronym means "Sleep Polyphasically As Much As You Like," and refers to taking 20-minute naps as desired throughout a day, and getting no other sleep. An experimenter writing under the name "Rasmus" lived on this schedule (and named it), averaging 7–9 naps per day, for over 18 months. A few others appear to have succeeded with it as well, though no-one seems to disagree that it's tricky as heck to maintain without getting overtired and crashing.

"Tea Time" Biphasic

This type of siesta sleeping standardizes on a 5-hour (sometimes 4.5 or 5.5) core-nap, and a 1.5-hour sleep during the day. Since it involves a long sleep during the day and a long enough core that one doesn't really gain much time overall, I'm not sure what the appeal of it is—but "Your Mileage May Vary" is definitely the name of the game here, and you never know; this might be someone's ideal schedule!

Substituting One Schedule For Another

As I've mentioned, I don't believe that sleeping 6 hours at night with one 20-minute nap would be sustainable in the long run, due to breaking the 6-hour-waking-period rule. But it's used by polyphasers, not infrequently, as a one-shot: I do it when the world messes with me and I only get one nap; I know that if I sleep 6 hours that night, I won't be a zombie in the morning. BUT I'm not aware of anyone who actually does that schedule as a long-term thing, and if I try to keep it up I will get tired unless I either sleep longer, or get more naps.

Another thing about my use of this schedule is that, if I sleep 6 hours, I can take 1 nap, but I prefer two. (I am "good and polyphasic" now, and I have trouble staying awake longer than 6 hours or so without a nap, no matter how long I've slept. I also can't really sleep 45 minutes like a siesta-sleeper would; I wake fairly automatically after 20 minutes now.) However, the number of naps needed has some variance, as you can see from the Formula. This is analogous to the "7–9" hours of sleep that constitutes the typical Adult 8 Hours... some people tend to need more sleep and some less. I take three naps on my Everyman schedule successfully, but if I can get a fourth, I'll take it, and when I do 1.5-hour Everyman, I like to have five naps—but when I'm monophasic, I need about nine hours, too. I'm just one of the people who sleeps a lot. (Ironic, isn't it?)

And there are other possible substitutions, too. Some polyphasers seem to be able to comfortably switch between known-good schedules on a one-off basis, as long as one of them is the regular schedule, and that one is kept as strictly as possible for the most part. This generally works for Everyman sleepers much better than Uberman sleepers; but it doesn't work for all Everyman sleepers either—for some people, messing up the schedule is messing up the schedule, and means either being tired while re-adjusting to the correct schedule, or falling back into monophasic sleep[16]. For my part, as long as I have a good 5–6 days a week of my usual 3-hour

---

[16] Falling back into monophasic isn't an imminent risk for me anymore; after about the first year, my polyphasic schedule has been my "normal" one. But if I consistently can't get naps for a few days, I will crash for 8 hours at night, and have trouble sleeping for naps the next day, and want to crash the next night... so I can be *made* monophasic. I even tried going back, as an experiment—there's a section on that later.

Everyman schedule with no major shakeups, substitutions don't seem to bother me at all. I will occasionally sleep 4.5 hours at night when I've missed one nap during the day, or sleep a full 6 hours on a weekend just for fun. As long as I get the appropriate daytime naps, I don't seem to suffer any ill effects from the substitutions. If things are crazy or crisis-y, I will occasionally do a day of 1.5-hour Everyman, or even Uberman, with little more than a few yawns and some coffee. So they seem to be interchangeable for me, as long as it's not very often.

So those are the schedules. Maybe you see one that looks like it might work for you... but, you, with your individual life, should you be polyphasic?

Of course that's an individual question, and those always come down to gut in the end. If you prefer, you can ask your guts directly and make a shot at it; but personally I like to have as much information in my brain as I can stuff in there before seeing what comes out of the guts. For those who operate similarly, next up is a chapterful of questions to ask and answer to get started.

III. The Big Question: Should You Be Polyphasic?

Wanting To

There are people in the world who have no interest in sleeping less[17]. But the experience of being alive (what we call "having time") is, after all, the most basic and fundamental currency of our lives: If we had nothing else in the world, we would still find it precious. Giving someone more "experience of aliveness" is akin to extending their lifespan; **it's no small gift to be conscious for four hours more every day than you used to be. That comes to 60.8 days more living per year,** hey. Two months! That means that every six years, you've gained a year. And if you're on Uberman, gaining about six extra hours a day, you get 91.25 extra days—a whole extra quarter of a year. You gain an extra year of wake-time every four years, which means that if you did Uberman for 20 years, you'd be five years more experienced in waking life than the monophasic people your age. Weird, isn't it?

Of course, this is not extra time in the physical sense; you're not really going to live longer from being polyphasic[18]. And philosophically, a good argument can be made that sleep may be just as important to the experience of living as being awake (though it'd be an argument lacking in evidence—I try it, and some of its cousins, out in the section on Philosophy near the end). I'm not of the opinion that sleep is evil[19], or wrong, or stupid; only that it's not, in my experience, as good a use of one's life-time as being awake is. If it's possible to be awake more without incurring some other big penalty (like illness or sleep deprivation), then why wouldn't one want

---

17   I've met several... we get along, but I don't think we grok each other. ☺

18   Actually there's no science on this one way or the other. So maybe you will!

19   Okay, granted, I used to be of this opinion. But I was young and fiery, and I did things like go all winter without shoes so that I wouldn't get too "soft". If sleep is really the nemesis I imagined it was then, then, well, so are shoes.

to do it? And in that, at least some the people I talk to seem to agree with me, and want to do it too.

Yet... when I first adapted to Uberman, and my friend and I both succeeded in it, approximately fifteen other people all tried to adapt to it, and *they all failed*. Like us, they were in college; like us, they had people helping, waking them up and watching over them and providing stuff for them to do. But most of them didn't make it a week! Why not?

Obviously there are many factors in play. Here are the things that seem to matter the most:

Being The Right Person

"Should I adopt a polyphasic schedule?" is one of the most frequent questions I get. It's usually accompanied by a "but", as in, "I want to be polyphasic but—". Since wanting to is the first step, we'll start with that and move on to the "buts" later.

Wanting to in the philosophical sense I just spoke about isn't enough. Philosophically speaking, we all probably "want" to be and do lots of things, but many of them aren't worth the effort. Polyphasic sleeping is definitely an effort; probably as much of one as becoming vegan or taking up an athletic regime. Sleep is a pretty fundamental thing to change! So **first you need to figure out if you want the change enough to make it worth the effort**.

That means asking yourself some questions and getting some honest answers. None of the answers by themselves are a deal-breaker, but if more than one of these questions reveals a problematic issue for you, you should seriously reconsider any plans to become polyphasic, and if you decide to go forward with it anyway, expect some challenges.

Here are the questions, though there may be others that can also be helpful:

1. **Why do you want it?**

   What's your primary reason? Is it powerful enough to be worth spending either several incredibly long days slapping yourself to stay awake, or several weeks feeling like you had half a night's sleep[20]? Think about what it feels like when you skip a whole night's sleep, and then double that and drag it out for a week—that's a good general image of what you'll feel like while you're adapting. Is the reason you want to be polyphasic compelling enough to be worth that?

2. **Do you have a reason other than wanting to try it out?**

   If your reason above is "because it's cool" or "I just want to try it" or "I want to see what it's like", think hard: Most people do much better if they have a compelling reason, even if they don't think they need one. If you don't have a compelling reason, can you create one, or do you really think you can motivate yourself sufficiently without one?

3. **Does self-discipline come naturally to you?**

   If not, you may (probably will) need to take extra steps to help you succeed. If you've never had to really discipline yourself, you may want to study up on some methods for doing that before attempting to change your sleep schedule drastically. Discipline is a habit, which means that once you "have" it, you'll fall back on it by default, and that's why it's important—because you will reach a point, at least once during adaptation, where you simply can't exert rational power over yourself anymore. Rationality can be a powerful force, but very rarely is it more powerful than your brain/body in full-on survival mode. When you reach that

---

20 Which one depends on the schedule you choose, obviously. It shouldn't be overlooked, though, that whichever schedule you pick, if you mess up during your adaptation, you could be in for both. (More about the Adaptation process in the next chapter.)

point, the only things that will keep you on schedule are a) someone else or some external thing forcing you to stick with it, or b) your habit of being disciplined.

4. **How are you with physical discomfort?**

If you can't stand feeling dizzy, spacey, tingly, dry-eyed, achy, weak, nauseous, stupid, and generally like you've been hit by a bus and then buried in peat moss, you're going to fold up, probably during or after day two. It takes a certain skill to let your body's discomfort be a bit separate from you, and without that skill, adaptation will be very, very difficult. If you don't have the skill and want to learn it, I suggest getting tattoos (piercings don't work; they happen too fast) ...or being pregnant for ¾ of a year and then giving birth. ☺

5. **How are you with mental discomfort?**

Besides the zombie-like levels of intelligence you'll possess for a few days during adaptation, it's also common to experience other psychological effects when deprived of sleep. Your brain is a survival machine, and it panics when it feels threatened, which it will when it suddenly stops being able to get the sleep it's used to (and until it gets used to sleeping on the schedule you give it). For a short time, you will probably experience doubts, mood swings, possibly some depression, maybe some psychosomatic physical symptoms, and quite likely a few hallucinations. Like fasting or any other extreme physiological challenge, adjusting to a polyphasic schedule means being able to beat your own brain at the game of controlling your body. It's not easy, but the feeling of victory is amazing. (And there are other rewards too, in this case.)

6. **How are you with people thinking you're a weirdo?**

This can range from funny looks to being publicly called a lunatic and told that you shouldn't be allowed to look after yourself if that's the kind of crap you're going to do... it can be mild or severe depending on your lifestyle and social surroundings, but it never stops, really, for as long as you're on the schedule. Also, are you okay with occasionally being cornered and asked tons of questions by people you wouldn't normally talk to? (It's taken me a while to get used to that!)

7. **How much do you need company?**

    One effect of polyphasic sleeping is that you tend to spend a noticeably higher percentage of time being by yourself. You're awake more often when other people are asleep, and sleeping during some of the time they're awake. Make sure your family and social selves (and companions) are okay with that. (If you get lonely and have a friend or partner who'll do this with you, that can be great... but if you like being alone, be careful of having anyone adapt with you, because you'll probably be seeing them a lot!)

8. **Are you punctual?**

    There's a massive amount of scheduling and timing involved in being polyphasic (compared to "regular" living, where your schedule is typically just determined by your activities, most of which assume a monophasic lifestyle). It's harder (i.e. crazy strict) while you're adjusting, but you still have to do some kind of scheduling for pretty much the whole time you're polyphasic. If you hate clocks, hate planning your activities, or are always behind-schedule and late getting places, you may want to either reconsider polyphasic sleep, or work on your punctuality first.

Lifestyle Contraindications

Okay, so let's assume you've decided that you're the right kind of person for this. There are still obstacles, unfortunately—some of which can be overcome, and some of which, sometimes, can't. The general rule from the last section applies here too: If more than one of the following is an issue for you, you may really want to reconsider, because being polyphasic could be very difficult for you. Having just one of these obstacles is usually workable, though it's still good to know what your obstacle is, because it gives you an idea where you're going to put the most work into adapting to and living on a polyphasic schedule.

1. **Do people depend on you?**

    By which I mean, do you have children, elderly relatives, or others who need you to be available on a drop-of-the-hat basis? Polyphasic sleeping can be a tempting idea for overworked mothers and caregivers, but the problem with sleeping much less is that you capital-n Need the sleep you do get. If you're going to be woken up from your naps, you simply won't be able to adjust, no matter what. (You also need enough help or time off to be a zombie for a few days while you adjust initially, of course.) However, if you can be assured of not being woken at all during your adjustment, and infrequently after that, then it can be worth a shot.

2. **Do unreasonable people boss you?**
Jobs can fit with polyphasic sleep-schedules just fine, but it depends on whether you can get a little freedom in your daily grind to take your naps. If you work on a factory floor with someone monitoring what you do every minute and sending you memos about cutting down on the duration of your bathroom breaks, then polyphasic sleep probably won't work for you. (That is, unless you work part-time, or your hours are short enough and/or breaks spaced right so that you can sleep at least once during the day, which even the most forgiving Everyman schedule will require you to do.) You can also try convincing your boss(es) that letting you have a nap is beneficial (because it is! See the Appendices for sample arguments to bosses).

3. **Do you like to party?**
Sure, polyphasic sleep makes the "rock and roll all night and party every day" dream look tantalizingly achievable, but unfortunately the two pursuits are usually incompatible. Once in a while doesn't seem to be a problem (or at least it isn't for me, but I don't tend to overdo it), but I've never seen a regular partygoer also manage to be polyphasic. Firstly, partying doesn't lend itself to taking a break precisely at X o'clock to get your nap (no matter who is currently hitting on you, talking to you, picking a fight with you, throwing up on you, etc.). It can be difficult, if you're "out" a lot, to find good and safe places to sleep; and even if you do always have a place to sleep, calming down from partying-mode into nap-mode, and then getting up and back into party-mode, is just too much of a jump for most people's systems. Also, alcohol and polyphasic sleep don't get along well; a glass of wine or a beer here and there doesn't seem to pose a problem, but getting really drunk will absolutely make

you oversleep, so if you like to drink very often, I would say don't even bother with polyphase[21].

4. **Are you on a very strict diet?**

It's not impossible to maintain a strict diet on a polyphasic sleep schedule, but it definitely is harder. For one thing, sleeping less can change your metabolism (the jury is still out on how, though the effects do seem to usually be mild, which is why it's only a known problem if you're on a strict diet), and if your diet relies on prescribed amounts of certain things, you will probably need to change those amounts to account for needing more energy. Also, if your diet is very "bare bones"—i.e. low-calorie, vegan, macrobiotic, etc.—then you may have trouble with the adjustment period, which is hard on your body anyway. (Nobody's ever gotten seriously ill[22] or injured as a result of the sleep-deprivation involved in adjusting their sleep schedule that I know of, but I do know that people with stricter diets seem to have more trouble maintaining enough energy to function[23].) Also, making two major changes at once is almost impossible, so don't decide to become polyphasic and go vegetarian at the same time, for instance.

5. **Are you ill?**

This sort of goes without saying, but if you have a chronic or long-term illness, or are currently sick with anything, you shouldn't even be thinking about messing with your system this way, at the very least not without the input of a doctor. A doctor will probably tell you that your body

---

21 I realize this technically isn't a word, but I've gotten used to using "polyphase" and "monophase" as shorthand for polyphasic- and/or monophasic sleep. If it bothers you, I apologize, but not too sincerely since I'll probably keep doing it ☺

22 With the exception of people who don't successfully adapt AND don't quit trying, therefore keeping themselves sleep-deprived for a stupid long time. I'll repeat myself about this somewhat, but this is why attempting polyphasic sleep, if you're going to do it, needs to be done *right* or not done!

23 After I'd been polyphasic for a year, I started experimenting with 24-hour weekly fasts. It wasn't horrible, but after a few weeks I had to make some changes, since the fasting was running me out of energy and I wasn't sleeping well. A 24-hour fast isn't really a big deal – but it's enough to affect a polyphasic schedule.

needs all the sleep it can get in order to heal or maintain your health, and I find little reason to argue, there. When I'm sick with one of the usual winter or sinus things that go around[24], one of the first things I do is sleep my butt off for a day, and it really helps me heal. In fact, a side-benefit of polyphasic sleep that I've experienced is that sleep is much more healing than it used to be. When I routinely slept 8 hours, sleeping in was useful but not magic; now that 4 is the norm, sleeping for 6 or 7 is amazingly restorative. I can't imagine restricting your amount of sleep while you're ill, but different illnesses function differently (some illnesses, for instance, actually benefit from fasting, which is also somewhat counter-intuitive) – so in the end, it comes down to asking your doctor and being responsible about it.

6. **Are you uninterruptible?**

Being polyphasic does sometimes mean having to put down what you're doing, sleep, and come back to it. If you find this incredibly difficult or impossible, either for personal reasons (you're autistic or have OCD, or you just hate being interrupted, or you're terrible at picking things back up after you've put them down) or for external reasons (you're a surgeon, or you conduct interventions or run a suicide hotline, etc.), then you will probably have trouble with polyphasic sleep. Then again, if your activities tend to interrupt your regular sleep anyway, you may benefit from polyphasic sleep, where you can recover (somewhat) with a nap rather than go a whole day being tired. (You probably want to stay away from Uberman, though, where missed or fudged naps can really wipe you out.)

7. **Are you crazy busy... enough?**

A polyphasic lifestyle can mean a lot of boredom if you don't have enough to do to fill all that time up. If you already spend some time every day wondering what to do next, then adding on 4–6 hours to each day is probably just going to drive you insane. While you can use some of your

---

24   I get these less often now than I did while monophasic, but that may be attributable to other positive changes I've made to try and take care of myself better—eating better and using a neti pot, for instance.

newfound time to relax and have fun (for some of us, it's the only reason we ever can), you can't use all of it, or even most of it, that way. (For one thing, if you tell your body that it's 2 ᴀᴍ and you'd like to relax now, it usually says, "Okay, let's go to sleep!") Ask yourself honestly if you are, or can be made, busy enough to use an extra 1/3 of a day, every single day. If the answer is no, you're probably better off just learning to manage your time more efficiently, than picking up a polyphasic schedule.

8.   **Are you loud?**
Depending on your living situation, polyphasic sleep may mean a lot of time being awake and being quiet, because other people are sleeping. Ask yourself if that's okay, and if you can stay occupied (not watching-TV occupied, but really occupied) while maintaining the level of noise-control you need. You can also plan things to do out of the house during key quiet-requiring hours, but that can be difficult or impossible depending on where you live.

IV. Preparing to Become Polyphasic

Time for the nitty-gritty. You've decided that you want to adopt a polyphasic sleeping schedule; now, how to go about it?

The preparatory steps are very important, in my opinion, in terms of ensuring your successful adaptation to a polyphasic schedule, and I suggest you do all of them if at all possible. That said, it would be disingenuous of me to claim that preparation is "everything", or that it's impossible to succeed without it: When I adapted to Uberman the first time, I literally heard about the idea one day, decided to give it my best try the next day, and got started on the first day I could fit it into my schedule. The only preparing I did was to make plans with a friend for help waking up, and to make a Big Fat List of things to do with the extra hours on the first couple days. So I can, and will, say that if you do nothing else, do something like those two things!

But every adaptation since, and every one I've talked through with other people, has been greatly helped by taking the following steps:

Researching

You're already doing a very important prepatory step: RESEARCH. Knowing about polyphasic sleep, what it is and what you want from it, and what to expect from the transition and afterwards, enables you to anticipate and plan, and to spot when something isn't working right and correct it. Besides reading this book, you may also want to follow some other adaptation stories in blogs or discussion groups, if you want a better idea of "what it's like"; and if you're scientifically minded or have a special concern, such as about a health condition, you may want to do additional research for that as well. Be warned: the pickings are slim when it comes to "actual studies" that show much about polyphasic sleep, because there haven't been very many studies done specifically on polyphasic sleepers. Quite a bit is known about naps and sleep-deprivation in general, though, so those can be useful places to start. Some additional resources for Research are given in the Appendices.

Deciding on a Schedule

Once you've done some research on polyphasic sleep, determine which schedule you want to adapt to. Picking a schedule that's right for you and your lifestyle will help save you the agony of an unsuccessful adaptation, so choose carefully. With a decision of this size, I find it's always a good idea to make, at the very least, lists of all the "pros and cons". Polyphasic sleep will affect nearly everything about your life in some way, so you want to make sure you consider the big picture.

Here's a useful hint for choosing a schedule: *If you have to heavily customize a schedule to get it to work around your life, then it's not a good one to start* your adaptation to polyphasic sleep on. Why the Uberman, Everyman and Dymaxion schedules work is still something of a mystery, and while it seems likely that other schedules built on similar formulas should work, testing them should be left to people who've already successfully adapted to polyphasic sleep in some form. When you're going from monophasic to polyphasic, you have no frame of reference for what it feels like when a polyphasic schedule is working. By modifying a schedule too much, you risk failing, either because the schedule you picked simply won't work that way, or because you have no way of knowing when it is working and so you quit for the wrong reason. Either experience would be miserable, so why go through it? If you're adapting from a monophasic or biphasic (siesta) schedule, *pick a known polyphasic schedule to try, and aim to make as few "customizations" to it as possible*.

Also, don't fudge the details because something "sounds better" or more likely to work. A common example is the 20-minute duration of the naps: Many people arbitrarily or emotionally decide to make it 30, or 40 minutes, thinking that this will make the schedule easier to adapt to. In fact, it will make it almost impossible to adapt, and 20 minutes really is the most optimum time to start with. Don't make changes "just because"; and if you really want to make a change, try asking some other polyphasers first to see if anybody's tried it, and what the results were.

Scheduling

Once you've picked which schedule you think is for you, write down your sleep schedule, noting activities that have to take place around it, such as work or classes. *Aim to have all of your sleeping happen at the same time each day.* If you're choosing an Everyman schedule, you can allow for some sway in the timing of your naps, but you should still plan to get them in at the same time whenever you can, and **plan to spend at least the first two weeks keeping strictly to the schedule**. If you have to permanently move a nap farther than you should (or at all, on Uberman), say, an hour later on Tuesdays, then expect this to make you tired at that time[25], and plan accordingly. Having an uneven nap schedule may also make your adaptation period slightly longer, but if you stick tight to your schedule, you will probably eventually get used to the unevenness, too. **Whatever your schedule is, writing it down will give you a good visualization that you can weigh changes on and use for planning**—I strongly suggest it, at least in the beginning.

This is what one of my written-down schedules looked like (for Everyman3):

---

25   Maybe just for a while, until you get used to it; but you may also *permanently* get tired around that time—it depends entirely on your physiology and your schedule. Sometimes the effects of moving a nap can be mitigated by tweaking, which conveniently, there's a chapter on!

	Monday	Tuesday	Wednesday	Thursday	Friday	Saturday	Sunday
Midnight	Read or relax	Read or relax	Read or relax	Read or relax	Read or relax	Read or relax	Read or relax
1:00 AM							
2:00 AM				3-hour core nap			
3:00 AM							
4:00 AM							
5:00 AM	Writing	Writing	Writing	Writing	Writing	Writing	Writing
6:00 AM	Leave for work	Leave for work	Leave for work	Leave for work	Leave for work		
7:00 AM							Breakfast w/gran
8:00 AM				Morning nap between 8:00–9:00 am			
9:00 AM							
10:00 AM							
11:00 AM							
12:00 PM						Short nap before Taiji	
1:00 PM	Lunch	Lunch	Lunch	Lunch	Lunch	Taiji Class 1:00–3:30	
2:00 PM				Afternoon nap between 2:00–3:00 pm			
3:00 PM							
4:00 PM						Afternoon nap	
5:00 PM							
6:00 PM	Taiji class 6:00–7:30	Home from work	Taiji class 6:00–7:30	Home from work	Home from work		
7:00 PM	Play time	Play time	Play time	Play time	Play time		
8:00 PM	Kiddo's bedtime	Kiddo's bedtime	Kiddo's bedtime	Kiddo's bedtime	Kiddo's bedtime	Kiddo's bedtime	Kiddo's bedtime
9:00 PM	8:30–9:00 Evening nap	8:30–9:00 Evening nap	8:30–9:00 Evening nap	8:30–9:00 Evening nap	8:30–9:00 Evening nap	8:30–9:00 Evening nap	8:30–9:00 Evening nap
10:00 PM	Homework	Homework	Homework	Homework	Homework	Homework	Homework
11:00 PM	Homework	Homework	Homework	Homework	Homework	Homework	Homework

Now, this wasn't the first schedule I ever wrote, nor the last. I've included this version because it contains several useful things to notice:

- *I did have to move one nap*, for my Taiji class on Saturday. At first I tried to just make it later, but I realized after a few weeks that I couldn't do 1.5 hours of exercise while sleepy, so I added in a 10 minute nap before class to take the edge off. That worked, so I kept it. ("Micro" or very small naps don't work for everyone, and I don't recommend them while you're still learning to nap, because they'll probably just make you more tired. By the time I added this, I'd already done polyphasic sleep for quite a while, so I was already used to napping.) I point this out because it's the kind of "little adjustment" that many people have to make, when life gets in the way of having a perfect schedule. It can take several weeks or months to get it all just right, so don't be upset if at first you adapt, but there are still some times when you get tired. (As long as you *have* adapted. If you don't adapt, there's a problem; read the rest of this chapter for more info on how to tell the difference.) Aim to have to make as few of these adjustments as possible, but don't stress about a minor one.

- *I have an hour's sway (half an hour in each direction) in which to take my naps, because I'm doing 3-hour-core Everyman*. It's still a struggle to get them in on time, some days, if work is hectic. If I goof up a nap, I get tired, just like one gets tired from staying up late or not getting enough sleep on a regular monophasic schedule. **On a polyphasic schedule, though, you feel your lack of sleep more (because you're getting less sleep overall)**. It's very noticeable, especially if I miss a nap—within an hour of naptime, I'll feel like a monophaser who got shorted by several hours the previous night. (On Uberman, missing a nap made me miserable for most of a day; I'd feel sleep-deprived within half an hour, and it would sometimes take several regular naps to catch up.) You go from zero to sleep deprivation very quickly on a polyphasic schedule, because you're squeezing more rest out of less sleep. **So it's very important that your schedule is possible, and that you're committed to sticking with it**. ...I should note that some people have more room to scoot Everyman3 naps around—I've heard from several people that they had up to an hour in either direction—but in my case, more than half an hour and I get way sleepy.

- *I schedule in my relaxation time.* If you have the tendency, as I do, to "run until you drop" (or develop physical symptoms of being overstressed), then it's not a bad idea to designate some book, game, art, or stare-at-the-wall time. When polyphasic, it's even easier than normal for a person who tends to overwork to get going and keep going ...and going... and going...! However, while you're adapting, you don't want your relaxation time to be where mine is, late at night or right before a nap, when you'll be tired. Try to put it during the day, or in between naps, instead, so you don't risk falling asleep.

- *I left unscheduled time on the weekends*—it's important, at least to me, not to feel like every second of my life is predetermined. During unscheduled time I get to do whatever I want, and even though that sometimes means mowing the lawn or running errands, it's still "up in the air" until it actually happens. Otherwise I start to feel like I'm in an Orwell novel. Whether you do this or not is up to you, but I do advise minimizing "unscheduled time" during the first week or two of your adaptation. When you're tired, it's very hard to decide what to do next. It's much better to always know what you should be doing, so you don't have to think about it (because chances are nothing will sound fun, at times, except sleeping!)

- *I had to give up eating big lunches*, because eating too much before a nap makes the nap less refreshing and harder to wake up from. However, I couldn't get a nap in before lunch (sometimes I can, in real life, but I couldn't schedule it that way), so I changed my diet to include small, light lunches. This has worked fine, but it shows how sometimes changes other than sleep are necessary.

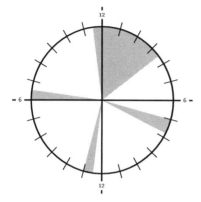

There are many other ways to keep a schedule, if you get creative: To the left is a scheduling-style based on a 24-hour clock, suggested to me by Eveline, a reader. (Thanks!) The colored sections are naps (this is a 3-hour Everyman schedule, obviously). This type of schedule lets you easily see whether your naps are evenly spaced, and would be great for scheduling other regular things like meals and exercise, as well.

You won't necessarily have to live on a schedule like this the entire time you're polyphasic. Some people will choose to, and others will loosen up or abandon their set schedules (except for the sleeping part) once they're adapted. What you do is up to you. I've done both, and overall I prefer having a schedule; but I've been polyphasic without one and it worked okay. They're a good idea to have while adapting, though, for the reasons shown above.

Your schedule doesn't have to be perfect, and you will make changes to it. But the better it is to start with, and the closer you stick to it, the easier and more quickly the adaptation period will go.

Strictness

One of the more frequent questions I hear is "how strict exactly does this have to be?" and "what happens if I miss a nap?" Those questions are answered indirectly in other parts of this book, but I'll take a second here to take them head-on, too.

Getting a nap late may make an *adapted* polyphaser tired for part of the rest of the day, but after a regular, on-time nap (sometimes it takes two), this usually dissipates. If you're already adapted, then missing or mis-timing one nap won't hurt your schedule—it'll just make you feel tired. **The danger, even after adaptation, is that, because you're tired, you'll oversleep a different nap, which will make it hard to fall asleep for another nap, which will make you oversleep another**

nap... and before you know it, your hard-won habit of napping at certain times and being fully awake in-between naps is in a shambles. Then you'll have to re-adapt, which, if you're already sleep-deprived from having missed too many naps and slept at too many irregular times, can be problematic too. Many poly-phasers who get out of the habit due to oversleeping end up having to go back to monophasic sleep for a while, to get rid of the sleep dep, and then re-adapt to their polyphasic schedule all over again. (Depending on several factors, re-adapting can be significantly easier than adapting the first time... or not.)

If you're still adapting, you may not feel as tired from having missed or mis-timed a nap, because your body isn't accustomed to relying on those naps yet. Oversleep-ing, or missed or late naps[26], while you're still getting used to your schedule may make you tired, or not, but they will definitely make it more difficult to sleep and wake up on time for a while afterwards. This is what's meant when polyphasers talk about "**extending your adaptation period**"—if you goof up naps in the first month or two, you make it take longer for your brain and body to get used to the new schedule. And you can't indefinitely drag out your adaptation without harm-ing your ability to sleep and get rest (see "Giving Up"), so it's really worth the effort to just make sure goof-ups don't happen!

Figure out how much leeway you need in your nap-times, and choose a sched-ule accordingly. Here are a few more general tips on choosing a schedule:

- Definitely don't choose Uberman unless you're confident that you can take your naps right on time, in all but the most extreme extenuating circum-stances. Missing sleep while on the Uberman schedule is really unpleasant, adapting to it requires perfect adherence initially, and failing to adapt to it is one of the most unpleasant things I have ever done. ::shudder::

---

26   It IS normal to not be able to fall asleep for some naps while you're adapting—that indi-cates that your body isn't using those naps for energy yet. You keep taking and waking up from all of them on time (whether you slept or not), and your body gets increasingly tired, and it can't stand it and it needs sleep, and that's how it learns to use the naps you're giving it regularly instead of the long sleep you're used to. That's really adapta-tion in a nutshell.

- Don't choose an Everyman schedule (with a core-nap) if you have to put the core nap right during the middle of the night (or whatever your natural sleep-period is) *and* you don't wake up well to alarms. People who do this often end up oversleeping endlessly (either by not waking up, or by falling asleep too early). Core naps are easier if you make either the time you go to sleep, or the time you wake up, one that naturally works for you[27].

- Whatever schedule you pick, take your time planning your adaptation. Very important! Try to do as much of the troubleshooting up-front as you can. **Don't rely on your "future self" to "figure out" what to do next: Your future self will be sleep-deprived**. Don't plan to make the tough decisions when you're going to be least able to do a good job—make them early, and firmly, and in as much detail as possible; and take steps so that you can remember them when you need to, even if you're barely functioning then.

Sudden, Mixed, or Gradual Adaptation?

When it comes to discussing methods of adapting to polyphasic sleep, there are numerous factors that could be changed about the process to produce what could be described as a "new method". I will focus on the different ways of introducing the new schedule, since there is much contention regarding which way is best; and unlike smaller factors, the way one introduces the naps may very well have an impact upon how much sleep-deprivation is experienced.

I do want to note, though, that in my opinion, the only difference, if there indeed is any, between one method of adaptation and another is probably the intensity of sleep-deprivation experienced. (And it may very well be a trade-off: If you experience less-intense sleep dep, you may feel it for longer—which isn't necessarily "easier". Some people may prefer a few really hard days to a few somewhat-hard weeks.)

---

27 Then again, you may not know what works for you until you try it. I wouldn't have known, for example, that waking up at 4 a.m. was easier for me than waking up at 5 or 6, until I Tweaked my early schedule (which had a 2–5 AM core nap. I was often tired before *and* after that nap!).

As long as the primary requirement of "replacing your current sleep-schedule with a consistently-applied and carefully designed new schedule" is met, adaptation should occur. Based on the process, it seems that you would incur some sleep-debt while you adjust, no matter how you do it. Changing how you start your new schedule might affect how quickly you adapt—or it might not. The jury's still out, frankly.

The three methods of adaptation I'm aware of are Sudden, Mixed and Gradual[28]. It's very difficult to compare them as wholes, because they've never been studied in a way that compares their effects while controlling for other factors, such as mistakes in the adaptation process, diet, and simply the differences between individual adapters—all of which might account for significant amounts, or even the entirety, of differences between polyphasers' experiences of different types of adaptation. But we can at least discuss what they are, and what the general idea of using them is, so let's do it.

In a sudden adaptation, you don't start out sleep-deprived[29]. For the first day, you aren't really sleep-deprived either; and you may not sleep for many of the naps. (It doesn't matter—the important thing is to train your mind and body that *this is sleep time*, so you lay down and attempt to nap for the full time no matter what.) By the second day, you're tired, and you may fall asleep for more naps, but will probably feel awful when it's time to wake up. By the third day, the sleep deprivation has gotten acute, and the body is starting to figure out that if it wants sleep, it had better get it during those naps, or it won't get it at all. You'll probably sleep for most or all of the naps that day, unless some of the symptoms of sleep-deprivation interfere, which isn't uncommon during adaptation either. You will break at least one alarm clock on this day, most likely. ☺

Doing sudden adaptations to Uberman, people almost always notice a marked improvement by day four or five, as it becomes easier to sleep for the naps, and

---

28 That's just what I call them; other people have different names, or no names at all, or don't care. Me, I like names. ☺

29 Unless you already are, for some other reason. Oddly enough, I've adapted both when I was already sleep-deprived from other factors, and when I wasn't, and I don't recall any difference that I might say was caused by that.

your system has gotten used to the fact that you wake up after twenty minutes, so it starts cramming more "rest" (however that works) into your short naps. You begin to occasionally wake up feeling refreshed and less tired. If you're adapting to Everyman, though, one of your naps is not the same length as the others, and this will probably delay your body's "figuring out" how to use the naps to its best advantage by several days. I and my partner, when we adapted to Uberman, experienced a lot of relief from sleep-deprivation on day four, and by day seven we'd stopped feeling tired at all. (Note that biologically, it almost certainly took a few more weeks before the schedule really "sunk in", and as evidence for that, we still heavily relied on alarms to wake us up for quite a while after that—it wasn't until we'd been on the schedule several months that we realized we no longer really needed an alarm.) ... When I adapted to Everyman though, it was a week before the sleep deprivation (which never got quite as acute as it did with Uberman) began to retreat, and two weeks before I felt "normal" (i.e. not tired) again.

So dropping into the new schedule suddenly, which I consider the "basic", most often-used approach, works by a) creating sleep dep at the same time as b) changing your available sleep-times to be the only ones your new schedule allows. After 1–4 weeks of "lag time", your body figures out the new schedule, and uses it to eliminate the sleep-dep and keep you rested from then on.

Mixed Adaptation

What I call a "mixed adaptation" is really a sort of pre-training for a sudden adaptation. The hopeful polyphaser begins taking one or more regular naps while still monophasic, and then after a period of time (usually a few weeks or more), initiates a sudden adaptation just like above.

The theory there is that part of what holds up the body's adaptation to a new schedule—creating the period of "lag time" where you feel sleep-deprived—is that it must "learn to nap", and that by learning to nap first, adaptation can be shorter. It's not a bad theory: For one thing, there is evidence that we do indeed "learn to nap", just like people learn to ride a bicycle and never really forget. The evidence is that polyphasers who go back to monophasic and then, months or years later[30] go back to a polyphasic schedule, find that it takes very little time, comparatively, to get back in the swing of falling asleep quickly and waking up after twenty minutes[31]. Former polyphasers who switch back to monophasic also seem to retain the ability to fall asleep quickly and wake refreshed from a nap, even while they're monophasic.

So that makes sense. The downside is that it's somewhat disingenuous to draw a direct line between "being used to napping" and "the adjustment process taking less time". There's no real evidence for that, or, as I said, none that controls for other factors. It's entirely possible, for example, that it's getting used to napping *within that schedule* that causes adaptation to happen, in which case extra napping beforehand wouldn't actually do much to shorten or lighten the discomfort of the adaptation process. In that case, all a mixed (or even gradual) adaptation does is to drag out the duration of the adaptation process.

My adaptation to Everyman—to reach the point where I was no longer sleep-deprived or having trouble staying alert the whole day—took a little over three weeks. That's on the longish side of normal, as I understand it. Then again, I failed at adapting to Uberman shortly before I decided to try Everyman, and I didn't take a break between the two, so I may have still been sleep-deprived when I started adapting to Everyman. ...But wait. If going through sleep-deprivation is part of the adaptation process, then maybe being sleep-deprived when you begin will make it go faster...!

That's the thinking, or some of it, behind the third type of adaptation:

---

30   Six years, in my case.

31   Which doesn't necessarily translate into a shorter adaptation—see the section on Forming the Habit—but it can mean less sleep-dep, since you can sleep more during your naps.

Gradual Adaptation

Frequently, the idea of "adapting gradually" is raised as a possible way to lessen the discomfort of adjusting to a polyphasic schedule. People who've done it tend to come up with some plan to "transition" from their current schedule (usually monophasic) to their chosen polyphasic schedule. As expected, this can be even more complicated to plan than a Sudden adaptation.

There's no compelling reason to think that gradually adopting your polyphasic schedule over a period of days, as opposed to starting it right away, will eliminate the sleep-deprivation part of adapting. It may reduce it, but if so, I think it probably does so at the cost of making the adaptation take longer. The most likely way one adapts to the new schedule is by being on it, not by being off of your existing one. However, until there's real data comparing the two, that's just as much conjecture as anything anybody else says.

The question of whether a longer period of moderate sleep dep is better or worse than a short period of holy-cow-wonkiness will remain in discussion for a long time, I predict. But there definitely is one downside to adapting gradually: It leaves more room for mistakes, and since you're going to be in the adjustment period longer as it is, you won't want to extend it even further by messing up. So if you choose to attempt this route, plan carefully!

Other Items on the Pre-Flight Checklist

Here are a few more things that can really help your adaptation. I strongly suggest making sure you have every one of these in place before you start—collectively, these items are the single biggest thing, besides research itself (and an iron stubbornness), that seems to make the difference for people between adapting and failing to adapt.

So, yes. These are suggestions, but very firm suggestions. Hence the checkboxes, which I think serve as a nice typographical passive-aggressive hint; don't you? ☺

☐ The Big Fat List

This is your best friend, and one of the things I credit the most with getting me through my adaptations—I even make (a smaller) one whenever I get off-schedule and know I'm going to be tired for a night or two while I straighten things out. The BFL is a monster list of everything you can think of to do with your extra time while you're adapting. No matter how tightly you schedule your days, you're 99% likely to have extra time. On Uberman, it can seem like endless extra time at first, so to adopt this polyphasic schedule, you'll want a really big list[32]. Don't forget to include some:

- items that can be done specifically at night, which may involve being quiet or not having much light;

- items that don't require much intricate thinking or coordination, since you'll be sleep-deprived for some of this; and

- items that keep your body moving, because sometimes it's flat impossible to stay awake without moving around when you're sleep deprived.

That's not to say you can't or shouldn't put "Learn Japanese" or "practice flamenco guitar" on your List; only that you should make sure to also include things you can do when you must be quiet, or when you're not at your best, physically or mentally. Also, while one big undifferentiated list is fine, it's also a good idea to set aside some "major undertakings" to accomplish (such as "dye all my friends' hair", "clean the garage" or "watch the entire Ring Cycle on TV"[33]), especially on nights two, three, four, and maybe five too. You don't want to be stuck wondering what to do next when you're extremely tired, because guess what you'll probably decide to do?

Also, think about what you want to do with your extra time in general, and incorporate some things into your Big Fat List that are good habits to start with. If you want

---

32 To give you an idea, when I adapted to Uberman, my list was over 80 items long... and I did all of it in about three days.

33 Assuming high opera would keep your interest that long. Then again, Wagner is not to be underestimated!

to spend your evenings doing martial arts, then why not load up your BFL with workouts and practice (both difficult and I-can-do-this-sleep-deprived easy)? Many people start out with grand ideas for using their free time, but then develop early bad habits of spending it all playing video games—which, if that's what you want to do with it, is fine; but if you start with that for your adaptation, it's going to be hard to switch to a new habit later.

Here are some of the specific Big Fat List items that really saved my butt, through both adaptations:

- **Cleaning** is probably the single best one, in my opinion. Organize the sock drawer. Re-arrange all the books. Scrub the corners of the room with an old toothbrush. De-tarnish all the silver. Dust the ceilings. These are all easy things to do when you're brain isn't working too well, they keep you moving, and they have the bonus of giving you a sense of accomplishment—look what you did with that extra time! Wow! Add some music for a little extra stimulation, and it can be a pretty fast way to spend the time.

- **Correspondence** is also pretty good, because writing letters, preparing cards and little presents to mail, and making phone calls is relatively entertaining, and being engaged with others (even indirectly) will distract you from feeling tired and/or crappy. Use some of your time to catch up with people you've lost touch with, or owe some kind of attention; again, you'll feel good about it, too.

- **Walking** comes highly recommended, especially at night, if you live in a safe area. Fresh air and brisk walking can really help wake you up, and if you're at the stage where you're having trouble sleeping for your naps, it can help tire you out right before a nap, too. (It helped me out so much during my first adaptation that, when I planned to re-adapt, I made sure to do it during the summer so I could walk at night!)

- **Cooking**, if you like to do it or want to learn. Be careful though; some polyphasers have gained weight while adapting, because eating is a good way to rouse yourself, and the smell/presence of food will help keep you awake.

(Just make sure you're around mostly healthy food. Being awake longer, it's okay to eat a bit more, as long as it's not a bit more junk!) Also, be safe: don't make flambe at 3 AM on day three!

- **Projects** that are sitting on your "perpetual to-do list" can be great ways to fill the time, but look out for two things: One, what specific activity does the project require right now? If it's at a stage where it needs two hours of Internet research, then 4 AM might not be a good time to do it. Second, don't be vague or you'll talk yourself out of it, or work on it at the wrong times. Make sure you write down what exactly to do, not just "work on that project".

- **Being Social** can help, as long as you're a) able to leave the social situation precisely on time to get your nap, and b) staying sober. If you've got a friend who wants to hang out with you at 2 a.m. though, that can help a lot. (Especially if you can talk your friend into sticking around while you nap, and helping make sure you wake up again.)

- **Exercise** gets tossed around a lot as a good stay-awake activity; personally I'm ambiguous about it. I love to exercise, but I've never had much luck talking myself into working out when I have that run-over-by-a-train feeling that accompanies parts of adaptation. And you definitely don't want to drastically increase your exercise regimen while you're adapting to a new sleep-schedule – your body can only take so much at once! But the occasional jumping-jacks or their equivalent do wake you up. Done moderately, and especially if it's something you enjoy, exercise can really help you, not only to stay awake, but to feel more alert and less like you've been sat on by a hippo.

- Lastly, feel **free to get weird**. Here's one I didn't tell anybody about at first, because (at least for a while there) even I didn't want to admit to being this weird. But heck, it worked (so well that I put it on my BFL the second time), and you bought the book, so you deserve to know about it. ☺ ...Sometimes being tired, especially for a solid week straight, becomes emotionally exhausting; you get sick to death of telling yourself not to think about it, not to act on it. And everyone (in my experience) who goes through this hits a point, or several, where you just feel like you can't do it anymore. When it was nearly morning of Day Three[34] of my first Uberman adaptation, I hit that point: I just couldn't take it anymore, and I certainly couldn't take it quietly. So I stood up in my dorm room, where I'd been trying to do something or another to stay awake, and shouted, "I'm [bleep]ing sick of being tired! I feel like my brains are made of Jell-O and melting down into my shoes! I feel like a zombie took a crap in my head! And why the heck are my arms tingling; what possible evolutionary good does *that* serve?" And so on. I ranted and raved pretty much straight through until I had to go to class, and lo, I felt tons better. So if all you can do is think about how tired you are, use it—get excited about it: pace around, wave your arms; do the mad-composer thing, the Cyrano thing (if you have something like a sword, heh), or an interpretative dance. Sometimes when all that's left in your mind is exhaustion, the sense of exhaustion itself can become your fuel for a while: Just let it out!

☐ Motivational Assistants

Remember, don't rely on "yourself, later" to do important things—including reminding you why you want to keep doing this.

- Spend some time solidifying why you're doing what you're doing, and get it in writing if you haven't. Make sure to include things that may slip your mind later, like "I hate how waking up in the morning feels anyway" and "I'm always tired at 4 PM".

- Write prolific notes to yourself with the key points on them, and leave them in places you'll see them when you need them most: By your bed, near the couch, on the TV, next to the computer...

- Explain your reasoning to other people who may be sympathetic. Then you can call them later and say, "Remind me why I'm doing this!"

---

34 It might have been the same time on Day Two; I'm not positive. The end of the night of Day Two is a common place for people to hit the skids, but I seem to remember getting lucky, because I was out in public the night of Day Two. It was three, I think, that really hit me like a freight train.

- If there's anything you can do to make this a Serious Promise in your own mind—swear on it, dedicate the effort to a cause, write it in blood, promise your grandma, bet someone a hundred bucks you can do it—then do it.

☐ The Kill Switch

In order to tell yourself to "keep going no matter what", you need to put aside the worry that it really might be time to quit, that you might be getting sick, etc. The best way I know to do this is to **designate someone else to be your "Kill Switch"**, a person whose job it is to keep an eye on you and call a halt to the experiment if it gets out of hand. That person will have to be able to watch you be miserable and look like crap for a while without freaking out. (Hint: Generally speaking, your parents are a bad bet.) Educate the person about what you're doing, what symptoms are normal, and what your goals are. Maybe even give them this book! *Make sure they know that you may very well try to talk them into letting you quit*, and set up some concrete instances of things that should make them worry, so they have some objective benchmarks. Make sure they know that it's normal for acute symptoms to continue for a week (Uberman) or two (Everyman). Then, let *them* worry about whether *you* need to quit, and don't you even consider it!

☐ Backup Alarms

These are an absolute necessity. Note that it says "backup alarm**s**"—two will work if one of them is really hardcore, but three is better, and five or six never hurts. Here's what I know about alarms:

- What wakes you up the best differs by person, so give it some thought, but in reality "what works best for you" matters more later on: During adaptation, you want to focus on quantity. Why? Because you're sleep-deprived, and so you're going to sleep through anything at times. The more mechanisms you have in place to wake yourself, the better!

- Do stagger alarms, but keep in mind your goal is to get up on time, not half an hour late after you've shut off six alarms. You are training your brain here; consistency and precision are key. Try to make your first alarm something that, unless you just sleep right through it, will compel you to wake up completely, and aim to never have to use your backup alarms. (You will, but the point is to *think of them as emergency backups only*.) Or use backup alarms to make you move around—set them all for the same time, but put a few in your room, one in the hall, two in the kitchen... by the time you get done shutting them off, hopefully, you'll be away from your bed and somewhat awake.

- Whatever else you have, make sure to have *at least two kitchen timers*. Aim for loud ones and, if possible, ones that aren't too easy to reset. These are highly portable[35], awesome alarms for use as backups or when sleeping away from home; and they can also function to remind you when it's naptime—just set one for the next naptime when you first wake up. A good cellphone alarm can take the place of these, but though I love my cellphone alarm, I still like to have a few timers on hand.

- The single most effective method of waking up when you're sleep deprived is probably to *have someone wake you*, especially if they put something in your hands that needs doing. (My awesome co-conspirator in the original Uberman experiments used to pop open a can of Coke and hand it to me, and I just couldn't go back to sleep when there was someone in my room and I was holding a full can![36]) The telephone also wakes many people (including me) reliably – I'll stand up and go answer it, even if I'm dead out... even if I don't wake up until some ways into the conversation! These two methods can be tough to arrange, but if they work for you and you can get them, especially for some nighttime naps over the first (and maybe second) week of your adaptation, I highly recommend it.

- Check and see if a wake-up call service is available to you—they're a weird perk that gets tacked onto the end of a lot of packaged services, like credit cards or club memberships. Or you could use something like www.wakerupper.com, which is one of several computer services that

---

35   Think "alarm going off that I stuck on the back of the fridge"

36   Our diets back then would make any carbon-based life-form wince—I'm certainly not advocating drinking that stuff. Anymore, all I use it for is to clean my car battery!

will call your house. Be aware that these may not be accurate to the very minute, so they may only work as backups and not main alarms.

- Don't forget your appliances! Anything that can be plugged into a wall can be put on a timer. Outlet-timers are cheap; I recently bought a two-pack at Ikea for something like six dollars. Your TV can be a good alarm, but don't stop there—one genius loaded his blender with the makings for a smoothie, and then plug it into a timer, so right when his alarm went off, the blender started up—noisy and requiring immediate attention, plus it produced food (cold, healthy food, even) that woke him up further[37].

- Another angle on that is the food alarm—not so much an alarm as a solid motivation to get and stay awake once your alarms have gone off. Using food (or similar preparations that you can leave alone for long enough to take a nap, but that then need your attention) can be risky, though; be careful you don't start a fire! But if you put something in the oven, take something out of the freezer and set it on the counter, put tea on to steep, or in any way start cooking something and then stop in the middle, it can really help you wake up (as long as your alarms are actually penetrating your consciousness—if you think they might not, don't risk it!).

- A variation on the Appliances theme is the ingenious idea of the "water clock"[38]. It takes a little geekiness to put together, but basically, if you can rig up a pump (on a timer), hose, and water source, you can be virtually guaranteed of getting up on time!

- I probably don't have to mention how computers can be useful as alarms; if you have one and use it enough for its presence to rouse you, you probably know, or can easily learn, seven or eight different ways to program it to wake you. If you can't though, don't worry about it; computers can't do much as alarms that can't also be done some other way. One thing people sometimes

---

37 Consider your luck, though: If it's like mine, the blender would tip over, and I'd get to wake up to a messpocalypse. Granted, I'd *definitely* be awake!

38 Great, now that I said that, I want to go get my dice and pencils. ☺

don't think of, but which works especially well on computer-centric people, is to rig a computer near you to turn off when it's time for you to get up. The subtle click of a PC suddenly powering down rouses me like a fire alarm!

- "Sleep tracks" are quite popular – these are sound recordings, of the right length for your nap, typically of silence or white noise, followed at the appropriate time by something raucous to wake you up. A gentleman with the nickname "Placebo" made the first of these that I ever heard of, and I used one of his myself for a while, because it was convenient and effective as an everyday alarm—other people couldn't hear it, and the white noise through headphones helped me sleep in noisier places. (You can still find the sleep-tracks on his website; check the Resources at the end. There are also several other sleep tracks published now, so search around if you don't find what you need. And of course, they're not that hard to make, either—20 minutes of white noise or silence, followed by a gentle alarm, and then something really obnoxious and LOUD in case it doesn't work!) I didn't use a sleep-track during any of my adaptations, though, so I can't speak to its efficacy while going through sleep-dep. Also, keep in mind that constant white noise while you're sleeping may affect the quality of your rest.

Among the many, many reasons for adapting right the first time is the **reductive efficacy of alarms**: They all work SO much better when you're not used to them! If you start off right, then you'll only need your million-backup-alarms for a week or two, and the really hardcore ones (like hoses and blenders) for only a couple days.

When they're all "new" to your brain, they work great—but if you goof up and start over, they're not so new anymore, and it becomes harder to wake up to them. What's more, people who fail to adapt and "keep trying" a lot can even make themselves somewhat immune to alarms in general, which in turn makes adapting nearly impossible. I feel terrible for these people, because, while they want to be polyphasic enough to keep trying to adapt over and over (and that's no picnic!), the more they don't get it right and keep coming back to it, the less likely they are to succeed.

(That said, if you must make more than one attempt, be prepared to have to shuffle your alarm-configuration *significantly*. The brain is *mad* cagey that way.)

```
<Author Intrusion>
```

...SO, by now we should have reached the point where:

- You know what polyphasic sleep is (or if you don't, please send me a nasty email because I'm the world's *crappiest* writer)

- You know if you're the kind of person, with the kind of lifestyle, who may enjoy and/or otherwise benefit from a polyphasic schedule

- You've learned what the different types of polyphasic schedule are, and how to go about picking one that suits you

- You understand the basics of how long adaptation takes, and how it works (as far as we know)

- You know how to plan for an adaptation, and some items or actions you can set up beforehand to increase your chances of a successful transition

...Which sounds to me like you're ready to get started! The following section begins discussing the adaptation process, sleep deprivation, and knowing when you've succeeded (or not).

Onward, then!

```
</Author Intrusion>
```

V. Adaptation Part One: Initiating Adjustment

Adaptation is a mystery, mostly, to people who haven't done it. It's a little like a trial-by-fire (in fact some people want to attempt it for just that reason), and very much an exercise in knowing your mind and body... and besting them in an epic week-long "battle of wills".

Everybody's experiences differ: Some adapt with little fanfare, sending me comments like, "I was really tired on day three, but eh, no big deal!"—and some people really have to fight their guts out, like the amazing middle-aged woman I talked to who'd been on Uberman for a year and a half... it took her over five weeks of struggling to adapt, but she did it and never looked back. (Not that you should necessarily persist for five weeks—what she did worked, but it was risky for her health.) But there are typical and less-typical experiences, so it's not impossible to get an idea what to expect.

Note: Some people actually do better with big difficult tasks like this if they don't know the details of what to expect. If that's you, skip ahead to section VI, which is about knowing when you've succeeded or when it's time to give up, and tweaking your schedule after adjustment.

The adjustment period can be defined by three major tasks, each of which is critical for the adjustment to succeed:

1. Lay down on time for all of your scheduled naps

2. Wake up on time from all of your scheduled naps

3. Do not sleep during unscheduled times

There will be various challenges getting in-between you and those three goals: Some of them will be related to changing your lifestyle; some will simply require discipline; and some will require overcoming negative physical stimulus. Just remember the Zen Proverb: **The obstacle is the Path**. *The habit-forming parts of your mind/body that you have to fight in order to adapt to your new schedule are the same parts of you that allow you to succeed*, and for the new schedule to eventually become effortless!

One challenge of adaptation that's almost universal (and I only say "almost" because I'm cautious like that; it IS universal to my knowledge) is the experience—usually the most in-depth experience you've ever had—of sleep deprivation.

Most people have experienced mild sleep-deprivation, such as you get from staying up for a whole 24 hours or so. Acute sleep deprivation is a bit different. You won't feel the acute sleep-dep for very long while adjusting to a polyphasic schedule, but even getting through a couple hours of it can be a major undertaking.

Short-term sleep dep, even acute sleep dep, is for the most part not dangerous. (It can be if you, say, operate heavy machinery; but you're not going to do that, now, are you?) It's just like hunger: It's your body attempting to get you to fulfill its need. As with hunger, you don't want to live with sleep-deprivation in the long-term: that could be very unhealthy. In the short-term, though, both my experience and my reading back up the fact that it's generally harmless.

Due to the symptoms it creates, though, it's safe to say that for most people, sleep deprivation is really unpleasant. It's *supposed* to be unpleasant, just like hunger is: your system is trying to nudge (or kick) you into doing what it wants. That's why battling sleep deprivation is often likened to "playing chess against your brain". The survival programming in the mind/body is what makes you eat, sleep, stay warm, reproduce, etc. And that's what you're up against, when you decide to ignore sleep-deprivation symptoms so that you can change your sleep schedule.

Sleep deprivation is surrounded by a bit of mystery, as well. No-one really knows why we need sleep—the negative effects of not getting enough sleep are almost all directly tied to the sleep-deprivation mechanism. So in theory, if you could turn off the sleep-deprivation reaction, and just not sleep, that should work—or rather, we can't tell why it *wouldn't* work, because we can't, generally speaking, turn off sleep deprivation without causing other effects (i.e. with drugs). But there are people who've gone really long times without sleeping who've survived it; and even, like the Thai gentleman I mentioned earlier, who've gone years without sleeping and are apparently fine. Those people have usually had something happen to them that short-circuited the sleep-deprivation response. Then again, when I was in high-school, the prevailing wisdom was that without any sleep, after about two weeks you'd "go insane" and die. For some people that might be true (I couldn't find any evidence of it ever happening), but the weird part is that if that happened, it would be because the sleep-deprivation killed them[39], and not because lack of sleep did.

However, the goal here is NOT to ignore sleep deprivation permanently, or to stop getting rest. **The goal is to teach the body a different sleeping pattern, and once it learns the new pattern, sleep-deprivation symptoms go away**. This has been scientifically proven to happen, thanks to Dr. Stampi[40]: We *know* that adjustment to polyphasic sleep is possible, and that once adjustment happens, sleep deprivation ends. So don't let anybody tell you that being polyphasic is about being constantly sleep-deprived! They either don't know what they're talking about, or are doing it wrong.

The symptoms of sleep-deprivation go away when your body begins getting the sleep it needs again. In most cases, when we're sleep-deprived, we sleep long and hard and keep at it until all of the sleep-deprivation is gone. When adjusting to polyphasic sleep, we do something different: We give ourselves *only* the sleep we would get on our new schedule. Because that means sleeping for a much shorter

---

39   I should add that I was unable to locate any cases of sleep-dep killing people directly (as opposed to indirectly, by "being sleep deprived while driving" or something). Sleep-dep is intensely unpleasant and definitely not a good state to be in, but it's not, as far as we know, permanently damaging in and of itself.

40   See the "Resources" Appendix for more on Dr. Stampi and his study.

period of time than we're used to, at first, the sleep-dep symptoms get worse. You don't get any sleep at first, and then you grow tired enough that you begin to fall asleep for your naps, but waking up and staying awake until the next nap is hard— sometimes *very* hard. But as you continue to take naps and wake up from them on a predictable schedule, your body catches on, and catches up, and the sleep-deprivation disappears. I've experienced this many times now; I *promise* that it happens. It just requires sticking with the schedule long enough, and pretty soon you don't feel tired at all anymore.

Comparing Sleep and Food

I make, and will continue to make, a lot of comparisons between sleep-deprivation and hunger. I do this because they are the same type of mind/body process—a survival-mechanism. Getting through a few days of intense sleep-deprivation is a lot like fasting for a couple days (I've done both), and they are similar in terms of the mental and behavioral tricks that tend to make it easier.

But there is one major difference between sleep-deprivation and hunger that I want to point out, too: Food is actually necessary, as far as we know. Reports of yogis who live on sunshine and the smell of apples aside, we have good scientific evidence that without something like a basic supply of nutrients, the body will suffer per-formance losses, illness, and eventually death. On the flipside, though, there is no such known requirement for sleep. We know that without enough sleep, people suffer performance losses... due to the sleep-deprivation mechanism kicking in. We know that if someone simply tries to stop sleeping, the sleep-deprivation will get more and more acute until eventually it forces them to sleep. If they're prevented by an outside force from sleeping, they may die from one or more of the symptoms of sleep-deprivation, if they're untreated and get acute enough (though I'll repeat, I'm not able to find a case where sleep-dep was *definitely* the *sole* cause for someone's death). Or they may develop a mental illness; sleep dep has been known to cause a psychotic break in very, very extreme situations. (Then again, most of the time those psychotic breaks are happening in places where sleep-dep is part of a torture scenario, or something else which very well might give someone a psychotic break all on its own; so again, it's hard to say what the actual cause is, or that sleep-dep all by itself is to blame.)

So you could go without sleep forever, in the right circumstances. You may be miserable from sleep-dep, but you won't die from lack of sleep.

But with food, if you managed to turn off the hunger response (as people with certain illnesses sometimes find happens), you won't simply continue to survive without food—you'll die if you don't eat, whether or not your mind/body is pushing you to. Sleep is different. It makes sense to assume that any physical process that has a survival-mechanism backing it up is necessary[41], or at least useful, but at least as far as modern (published) science has gotten , there doesn't seem to be a firm answer for why we need to sleep, aside from "to keep away the harmful effects of sleep-deprivation". If you were able to turn off the sleep-dep, it's unclear what, if any, negative effects you would suffer from not sleeping.

But sleep-dep and hunger are, for whatever reason, controlled by the same mind-body *system*—the survival mechanism. This is the same mechanism that causes you to flinch away from danger, to fear the dark, to gasp for breath, and to pull your hand off of a burning stove. Outsmarting it is no joke—though it is, of course, possible. If you're going to "beat" sleep-dep (or hunger), though, you should understand this up front, and be prepared for a serious battle with yourself. (Some people find winning such battles really exhilarating—count me among them—and if that's you, strap on your best sword and get ready to be *really* thrilled with yourself at the end!)

How Much Sleep-Dep?

Adapting to polyphasic sleep, you will probably experience more-than-mild sleep-deprivation. Physical symptom-wise, it can feel as bad as, say, having a bad flu; but it won't usually be that bad for more than a few hours at a time. (You're probably aware of the concept of the "second wind", where someone who is sleep-deprived suddenly gains energy and feels fine for a while, then goes back to being sleep-deprived later. During the adjustment period, you will get multiple "second winds",

---

41   Though maybe not necessary for everyone—remember, there are survival mechanisms all over the place that back up the "need" to reproduce, but that doesn't mean every single person should or must do it.

meaning the actual acute feeling of being very sleep-deprived usually won't last more than a few hours at a stretch—it'll come and go.)

Again, to my knowledge, no-one has ever suffered a serious mental or physical injury from this level of sleep-dep *by itself*. But it's very important to take safety precautions, like not driving, being careful with things like fire and chemicals if you have to use them, and knowing when you're just too messed up to do something. There will be a few days, usually, where you're pretty useless—be prepared for that. But on a polyphasic schedule, you are giving the body an "out"—you are taking regular, predictable-to-the-minute naps, and it doesn't take more than a few days of really unpleasant sleep-deprivation before your mind/body figures out how to use the naps you're taking in order to get the sleep you need. (How exactly it does that is as mysterious, I think, as the benefit of sleep-deprivation as a survival mechanism.) I have seen no reason, in the years I've been doing and discussing polyphasic sleep, to be concerned about very harmful effects like psychotic breaks. **The sleep-deprivation in a polyphasic schedule should not last more than a few days, and restful sleep should begin to resume within a week, after which the level of sleep-dep decreases and then disappears**.

I know I sound like a broken record now, but I'll reiterate anyway: This is precisely why strictness and consistency is KEY. The more mistakes you make, the longer you drag out the sleep-deprivation, and the worse its impact on you.

The Mind/Body Survival Mechanism

What we call "sleep deprivation" is part of the mind/body's built-in survival mechanisms. As such, it is complex, and individual experiences of it vary, as does one person's experience at different times.

It's important to remember that what you're experiencing is the effects of a survival mechanism, and that it has a purpose, even though it may not be clear at times how exactly the process is working. *It helps to remember that much of what you experience as a physical reaction is also mental, created to spur your behavior in the direction of getting more sleep.* So if, for example, you normally crawl into bed when you feel depressed (or cold, or achy), then it wouldn't be surprising if you felt depressed (or cold or achy) as a result of a good dose of sleep-deprivation. Your body wants you to go to bed!

But, while much of the mind/body's sleep-deprived behavior makes some kind of sense, some doesn't. All living things carry old genetic data around that can become active at odd times, and countless environmental or other factors may be involved too—so don't get obsessed about finding the cause of every little symptom, either. If you do that, you're likely to get scared at some point, by a symptom you can't pin down or rationalize.

Do not forget that a survival mechanism involves both the body and the mind. When your goal is to stay awake and your body—including your brain—is feeling the effects of sleep-deprivation, your own mind will work against you.

Your mind is not an insignificant opponent—you might say it's your perfect nemesis. In a survival situation it becomes armed with direct control over your physiology. In order to bully, coerce, confuse, convince or lull you into sleeping, your mind/body might cause you to smell things, see things, think things, feel things (both physically and emotionally) ...it's not as bad as the freakouts you see in the movies, not at all. But if you're not ready for it, especially if it causes you to become anxious or scared, it can be a little hairy. As with actual survival situations, one important way to keep sleep-dep from overwhelming you is to **stay calm**.

Think of it this way: If you were stranded somewhere and fear was threatening to overwhelm you, you would want to force yourself to be calm, and you would benefit by reciting your goals to yourself—"Stay calm, find water, signal for help..."—and by focusing on what you can do *right now*, rather than what might happen later. When dealing with possibly-overwhelming sleep-dep, the same rules apply. **Stay calm, focus on your goal, take one step at a time**.

Besides educating yourself about the effects, and remembering your goals when it gets tough, you can also mitigate the negative effects of sleep-deprivation by being prepared ...starting by having a few generally-good-idea items on hand.

Good Things to Have on Hand while Sleep-Deprived

- Music, movies, books, games, or other media that make you feel upbeat, content, happy, pleasantly nostalgic or intellectually stimulated.

- Immersive activities that will distract you from thinking about sleep, or how miserable you feel: Video games are a big hit, as are night-time social activities like roleplaying games, poker games, pool... a hobby that really "sucks you in" works as well, but don't plan to be doing the same thing for hours and hours, since you'll probably bore or get burned out pretty easily when you're sleep-deprived.

- At least one room that you can light brightly and close the shades to, in case the darkness becomes disconcerting.

- Things that are calming, uplifting or invigorating to your senses—that smell, sound or look ways that will improve your mood and maybe give you some extra energy. The smell of oranges, oddly enough, helped to wake me up and lift my mood.

- A supply of pleasant hot or cold drinks that are not (too) caffeinated or alcoholic—if you've ever been curious about herbal tea[42], now is a good time to experiment!

- The phone, text, or IM number of an understanding someone who'll be awake during times that you may be alone and sleep-deprived (hint: the Internet is a wonderful place to find friends in other time-zones).

- Lists of reasons why you want to be polyphasic, and why it's important to only sleep exactly as your schedule dictates. (There are some sample lists

---

42   Tea is good for other reasons: Different teas have their own benefits (ginger will warm you up, for example), and there's a huuuuge variety of them. Also, tea takes preparation and maintenance: Getting a cup of tea will burn 5–10 minutes of unpleasant boring sleep-deprived midnight time, whereas opening a can only burns a few seconds.

and such in the Appendices, even.) It's not a bad idea to keep these where you would have to move them to get into bed!

Common Symptoms

It's normal, when sleep-deprived and especially during episodes of acute sleep-deprivation, to experience any of the following physical symptoms: Chills, body ache, dizziness, headache, dry/sore eyes, and falling asleep against your will, including while sitting or standing. You may also experience nausea, prickling or tingling sensations, or other physical events. It's also normal to experience mental/emotional symptoms, such as mood swings, irritability, auditory or visual hallucinations, confusion[43], feelings of helplessness or despair and a desire to give up.

Remember what you're up against: Your own mind/body, in survival mode. Knowing this will make the symptoms seem less scary and random, and you'll be better able to respond appropriately to each one. Sometimes you'll want to alleviate the symptom to make yourself more comfortable—with a warm shower, or eyedrops, etc. (just not sleep!)—and sometimes you'll find it best to ignore it and plow forward. Remembering what you're dealing with will also help greatly with the mental symptoms, especially when giving up begins to sound like a sweeter and sweeter plan: If you remind yourself that the feeling of wanting to give up is itself a symptom, you'll be less likely to give in to it. Staying aware of the nature of the problems—that they're caused by sleep-dep and normal and temporary—can also help you stay calm. Anxiety exacerbates almost every symptom, physical or mental. See the Appendix on Relaxation & Breathing techniques for more.

Remember, your brain is actively going to encourage, even try to force, you to change your mind about not sleeping. It will aim to make it miserable to continue, and at least for a short time, it will probably succeed! You'll need to have decided firmly, before beginning the experiment, to keep going in spite of any amount of

---

43   This one looks innocuous, but don't underestimate it... it can be really disturbing to realize that you can't figure out how to put your shoes on at the moment. The right way to handle it is to go do something else for a little while; when you come back to it, you'll be able to tie your shoes again!

misery[44]. It helps to keep reminders on hand of why you don't want to quit—sticky-notes, recorded messages, whatever you think will work. **Remind yourself that if you stick to your schedule, this part will be over soon**! Not only will your naps begin to make you feel more rested soon, but if it's hours until your next nap, remember that you'll almost certainly get a "second wind" in there somewhere; acute sleep-deprivation rarely lasts for very long.

Other Physical Symptoms of the Adaptation Period

The process of adopting a new sleep schedule puts your system under a pretty good load of stress, which can cause different effects in different people. Obviously if anything extreme happens, or if you think something's wrong, see your Kill Switch and/or doctor-figure. These other symptoms have been reported to me by polyphasers as temporary effects of sleep-deprivation:

- Increased or decreased appetite

- Tendency to feel cold; goosebumps—or alternately, hot flashes

- Dry eyes; periods of blurred or doubled vision

- Balance issues or vertigo

- Dry mouth or dehydration (make sure you're getting enough water, since lacking it can make many of the symptoms worse)

- Stiffness or muscle cramping (again, get enough water & vitamins)

- Tinnitus (ringing in the ears)

---

44 Tell yourself (loudly, constantly, in writing—whatever it takes) that no matter how much it sucks, you're going to do it perfectly for one whole week. If you do, and after a week you don't feel 75–100% better, then there's something very wrong with the schedule you're adapting to, or how. If you do feel better, but not fully, then remind yourself that it takes at least 30 days to become fully adapted, so don't start slacking off now!

- Weak immune system, especially if you're prone to such weakness (if you are, take extra steps to strengthen your system before and during—good healthy food, lots of vitamins, etc.—and make sure you don't start your adaptation when you're already feeling under-the-weather)

Can the Sleep Deprivation be Minimized or Shortened?

Sleep deprivation, while no fun, is an important phase in adjusting to any polyphasic schedule.

The sleep-dep is your brain "talking to you", telling you that it's no longer getting rest; and you're "answering" it by taking regular naps[45].

Your mind/body is very much a machine in some ways, and the way it works here is fairly predictable: Sleep-dep is the normal, first-line response. **When increasingly acute sleep-deprivation doesn't make you change, your brain will try another response: It will adjust** to the circumstances it's stuck with, and switch to getting the sleep it needs by adapting to your new schedule. (Why does your brain do this? The science is still a mystery, but if you think about how fundamentally adaptable human beings are, it makes sense that, given *some* predictable rest that it can use, the brain would get around to just using it, rather than staying sleep-deprived!)

When this adaptation works, you'll stop having sleep-dep symptoms—usually gradually, though once it begins to let up, the rest goes away quickly in my experience. (Sleep-dep disappears more quickly on Uberman than Everyman, I suspect because the perfect regularity of an equiphasic schedule is easier for the mind to adapt to.) It's the sleep-dep – having it and beating it – that makes polyphasic sleep work, in a sense[46].

---

45 Regular naps in a pattern known to provide the rest you need, once you adapt. As we discussed previously, just any old naps won't do it.

46 Some people claim that a more gradual adaptation can still work while minimizing sleep deprivation symptoms; I discuss that in the earlier section on Adaptation Methods. But the short answer is, "It's a long shot."

This, to say it again, is why consistent adherence to your new polyphasic schedule is so important: **If you respond to sleep deprivation by sleeping extra, then you're telling your brain that it doesn't have to adapt; that applying the right pressure will make you change back to the comfortable old habit of sleeping for long periods of time. If you give in (even once), your brain takes it as a sign that it should keep up—even increase!—the sleep-deprivation symptoms, since they're working**. It's imperative that they not work; that no matter what the symptoms, you sleep on your new schedule exactly. This will get your brain to give up on sleep dep as quickly as possible—usually within a few days—and resort instead to changing your sleeping patterns so that your naps give you the rest you need. **The more "mistakes", the more sleep-dep.**

That's not to say, however, that avoiding the symptoms of sleep-deprivation is impossible—it might not be. Maybe someday someone will figure out the perfect adaptation-method, one that puts just the right pressure in just the right places to change one's schedule without causing (as much) discomfort.

I rather doubt it, though, simply because the sleep-deprivation mechanism is so basic to our physiologies, and its exact expression differs so much among individuals. If you really can't stand sleep dep, though, you may want to keep an eye on polyphasic sleep research, just in case the answer is nigh. ☺

The Hard Part: The "Narcolepsy" Symptom

For most people, out of all the sleep-dep symptoms, the narcolepsy is the really tough thing to handle. Most people are lucky enough not to have experienced prolonged narcolepsy, though it can be a disease all on its own for some unfortunate individuals[47].

---

47   I refer to narcolepsy as a symptom, because the word is commonly used to describe *the state of falling asleep uncontrollably*, even when it's temporary. The disease "narcolepsy", which is what the technical use of the word usually refers to, is characterized by frequent uncontrollable sleeps, often ruining someone's life and/or requiring medication. Narcolepsy-the-symptom can also be a side-effect of some medications or other conditions.

During the course of normal sleeplessness, people will usually get sleep-deprived enough to experience narcolepsy as a symptom, and then they either fall asleep, or are kept going by some emergency or other heightened situation which overrides or blunts the narcolepsy. Unfortunately, you're unlikely to have, or be able to manufacture, enough emergency-like situations to get you through all the narcolepsy of your polyphasic adaptation. You will probably have to "tough it out" at least once; and for most people, that's a unique experience and a heck of a challenge.

So, narcolepsy is the fancy term for what's commonly, sometimes jokingly called "falling asleep standing up". But that's no joke—you really can fall asleep standing up. Or in the bath, or driving, or while stuff is on the stove… needless to say, **when you're experiencing this symptom** (which typically comes in hour-or-less-long spurts), **it's imperative to observe safety rules**, like you would if you were taking heavy painkillers.

- DO NOT operate a vehicle or other heavy or dangerous machinery. If you are in the middle of doing something dangerous, like driving, and you start to notice narcoleptic symptoms, *stop* immediately, take some of the steps listed here to alleviate the symptom, and *don't continue* until you're sure it's safe.

    - Remember that you're doing a one-time, special thing when you're adapting to polyhphasic sleep, and it's perfectly OK to need to take extreme measures, like calling someone for a ride home, or having to stop your car six times to get through the last mile, or take a day off work. It can be easy to feel awful about doing these things, but remember it's not permanent; you'll be hyper-competent again before you know it!

- For driving specifically, if you begin to nod off, do one or more of the following:

    - Open the windows all the way and crank the radio

    - Sing very loudly and enthusiastically

- Do "The Shuffle" (see the Cheat Sheet at the end on "Things to do when you're tired" for a description of this technique)

- Pull over, get out and take a short, brisk walk, run, or do jumping-jacks

- DO NOT "just keep driving" or try to "get through it"! Saving a little time is not worth having an accident!!

Also, while narcoleptic symptoms are typically worst at night, they can sometimes happen during the day as well. I always advocate being off work for the first few difficult days of your adaptation (typically days 2–5 or so), but if you do have to do sensitive things during this time, you'll want to keep a sharp eye out and take steps to alleviate narcolepsy as soon as you notice it coming on.

Alleviating the narcoleptic symptoms of sleep deprivation is not always possible—there will be short periods where your body is absolutely trying to fall asleep, right here right now. All you can do then is force yourself to stay awake until the feeling passes: By hopping into a cold shower, shaking your head or slapping your face, jumping or running in place, or taking a brisk walk outside, for instance. (Or—this one I thought was particularly smart—by holding dishes. One creative polyphaser told me about walking around his house carrying a big stack of dishes, which not only kept him from falling asleep, but guaranteed that if he did, he'd wake back up immediately!) I myself have stood next to a wall, letting myself fall into it and bump my shoulder (or head) as a way of jolting me back awake, for probably twenty minutes.

Almost every polyphasic adaptation involves getting to the point of needing to do things like that at least once—but don't worry; typically those spells are very short. (Unfortunately, they don't seem short.)

But fortunately, if you catch narcoleptic symptoms right when they're starting to creep up on you, there are things you can do that will often head them off before they get severe.

When you feel narcoleptic symptoms coming on, there are a few things you can do right away to try to stave off that falling-asleep-standing-up feeling, before it gets to the point where you're slapping yourself while blaring Star Wars on the TV as loud as it will go. The "early warning signs" typically include:

- Dizziness and a feeling of gently falling, or spiraling downwards (into sleep)

- Uncontrollable closing of the eyelids

- Heavy, difficult-to-move limbs

- A need or tendency to "curl up" your limbs

- Difficulty standing or sitting straight

When those things manifest, your body is trying to shut the lights off on you, so pay attention! Often, if you do one of the following things (or something like them) when you begin to feel this way, it will pass.

Note:

If you can't think of anything else to do, because your mind is blurry and there's nothing at hand, just keep standing/walking/etc. until you do think of something. As long as you keep moving, you should be able to avoid falling asleep.

Combating Narcolepsy Before it Sets In:

- STAND UP! You'll typically notice the above symptoms while you're sitting or reclining; the very first thing to do is get up and MOVE, no matter how much you don't want to. In fact, walking itself can be a good cure—just keep going until you feel better. Dancing works great too—but so does jumping in place, or even just standing and swinging your arms. Just move your limbs, and keep them moving.

- Make and eat a small meal or snack. Something that takes a little preparation, and/or effort to eat, typically works better than throwing a frozen burrito in the microwave. I used to cook a whole artichoke, and melt butter to dip the leaves in—by the time I was done making and eating it, an hour could have passed, and any nasty sleep-dep symptoms I'd been having were over.

- Pick up or put on a book, movie, or other entertainment that you find very interesting, which tends to engross you completely[48]. (Sometimes one you hate can be as effective as one you like, if you really hate it. Political media from an extreme opposite viewpoint of your preference can be very useful.)

- Begin a personal-care routine, especially one that you either associate with mornings or only do rarely. Just be careful if you're working with sharp things or chemicals! (I've hennaed my hair with great success for this purpose—henna is messy and tricky to work with, and the process takes several hours.)

- Change your clothes, and take some care picking them if you can. One thing that seems to work particularly well is to change into something that's not too easy to get into, and which you'd never normally sleep in, like formal clothes. (What the heck, do your hair/makeup/whatever too, if it helps. You're up; you might as well be pretty!)

- Take a cool or cold shower—*not a bath*, however, since the risk of falling asleep in a bath is too dangerous. Along the same lines, consider opening windows or lowering the temperature where you are some other way: Warmth contributes to sleepiness. (If you're having coldness as a symptom and you can't bear the idea of not being warm, though, try brisk exercise as a way to raise your body-temperature without encouraging sleep.)

- Talk, recite poetry, sing, or play a musical instrument (whether or not you can do it well): The concentration required to express yourself out loud will distract you from feeling sleepy.

---

48 I've heard that polyphasic adaptation is a great time to rent/borrow/buy an exciting book, TV series or other type of entertainment. (Or better yet, more than one.) And I can see the rationale, because I've gotten "sucked in" to new media and stayed up late just as much as the next guy. It's a good idea if that kind of thing engrosses you, but *take care sitting down*—putting in your DVD or picking up that book *while standing* may be a much better idea. Also, make sure you don't get *so* engrossed that you miss naptime!

- Court a little (just a little!) danger. Going for a walk at night if you're scared of the dark—or going to a cemetery or other "creepy" place—getting just a little bit of a scare on—is a fantastic way to wake up. Put on a very scary movie, even. Just make sure you don't scare yourself so badly that you can't sleep when it's actually time to!

- Make a phone call. Now is a great time to know someone in another time-zone!

Things that you don't want to do when you're feeling the onset of real falling-asleep-standing-up narcolepsy include flipping channels on the TV, reading magazines, surfing the 'Net, or just staring at a wall (which is probably what you'll feel like doing). In order to talk your body out of heavy-handedly pushing you towards sleep, you need to convince it that you're too busy right now, in a way it finds legitimate[49].

If you miss that golden opportunity, though, and actually start to exhibit narcolepsy—you awake with a start, in the middle of doing something, and it's only been a few seconds or minutes (you're having what polyphasers call "microsleeps")—then things get more difficult. But this will happen to you at least once; it does to almost everybody. Fending off narcolepsy once it's already happening is no fun, but don't give up! It doesn't last very long, and if you get through it you'll feel better in no time. (Remind yourself that *this is it*, this is the important part of the whole process, the point you've been waiting for. If you win this battle, things will get easier and start to work the way you want them to!)

The following tips should wake you up enough that you can go back to the previous list. For all of them, it's important that you follow up with something that'll keep you awake, like a meal or conversation. If you do any of these things and then go sit on the couch, you'll be back to square one! (Or as my friend used to

---

49   That means that different things work better for different people: Some people can snoz out while eating; others' brains could care less about being in the middle of a manicure. Fear is one of very few things that seems to work universally.

tell me, "Get up! We're going to be awake 22 hours a day—you'll have time to relax later!" ...And she was right; once we adapted I could relax plenty.)

- Stomp! Stomp, stomp, stomp. Lift your legs high and stomp—the jarring feeling of your feet landing hard will help, as will the balance challenge. If you know any martial-arts forms or drills, you're lucky, because practicing them is also an excellent way to back away from the edge of narcolepsy. Pick ones that include fast movements and some abrupt motions, but be wary of jump-kicks—you're not as balanced as you usually are!

- Similarly, hit something: punching bags are awesome, or substitute whatever you've got that's safe, like pillows.

- Stand near a sink or bowl of ice-cold water and splash yourself in the face, arms and neck with it repeatedly.

- Step into a really cold shower. (In your clothes, if you have to. Dealing with the mess and changing clothes when it's over will help keep you awake, too.)

- Go for a run or brisk walk, especially outside if it's cool out.

- Do jumping-jacks or another quick aerobic exercise. Keep going until you're out of breath, but don't push it too far, or you'll make yourself even more tired.

- Put yourself in as (physically) uncomfortable a situation as you can: if you can't sleep with lights on, turn them all on bright; if you don't like noise, turn everything up or put on loud headphones; if you hate the dark, go out in it ...when you feel a little more awake, go back to the previous list and find something sleep-unfriendly to do that's a little more comfortable; it'll feel like a reward.

- Do some advanced breathing exercises, if you know any. (Simple ones are usually relaxation-oriented and not a good idea! But if you're familiar with any energizing breathing exercises—Zen, Yoga and Taiji all have some—you may want to practice them until your head clears.) Beware of sitting or lying down, however—do standing exercises whenever possible.

Another challenge will present itself after you get through a bad sleep-dep spell, and/or fight off a bout of narcolepsy: The effort will wear you out! It's not uncommon to feel weary, drained, and generally crappy after having successfully navigated a period of difficult sleep-dep symptoms. Going to bed just sounds good on principle, even if you're not tired anymore. And of course, then eventually you do go to bed... and have to wake up 20 minutes later! (Note: Buy at least one extra alarm clock to compensate for the fact that you'll almost certainly break one at some point, out of sheer rage/hatred. For similar reasons, if you have a really nice alarm clock, maybe put it away until the first week has passed.) But all these things pass quickly, and if you keep your eye on the ball, the hard part will be over with before you know it.

Here is a short list of the things I personally found most useful in managing the sleep deprivation through my own adaptation-periods.

PD's Top Ways to Fend Off Sleepiness

- Shadow-boxing

- Dancing

- Singing

- Brisk Walking

- Reading aloud from favorite books/poetry

- Talking on the phone (while pacing)

- Sculpting, Painting, or other "messy" art projects

- Organizing drawers & closets

- Making smoothies or homemade juice

- Scrubbing not-often-cleaned places

- Going to the store (whatever's open)

- Making lists (of anything)

Also, don't forget that **for these ideas to be effective, you have to think of them at the right time**—which just so happens to be a time when your brain is functioning about as well as boiled cheese. I highly suggest WRITING DOWN a list (or five) of things to do when you're zonked, and putting it (them) in places where you'll see it (them) at the critical time. You can use the Tiredness Cheat-Sheet at the end of this book as a template, and add your own ideas as you think of them. (There are also a few more "extreme" and "weird" ideas on that cheat-sheet, just in case you really get stuck.)

Ack, I Can't Sleep!

Especially if you were suffering from insomnia before you chose to start a polyphasic schedule, you may notice that you can't sleep for your naps at the beginning.

It's a really annoying thing to have happen, to be unable to sleep when you've only got 20 minutes to do it in and you've been tired for hours. Almost everyone finds they can't nap during some of their daytime naps on the first, and sometimes the second, day, but for insomniacs (and sometimes for non-insomniacs too), it can be as long as several days before you get even one good restful nap. This isn't a bad thing; it's just another path to adjustment that the brain/body sometimes takes. You won't be any more tired than someone who's successfully getting 20 minutes of sleep and then waking up, trust me. Your mind and body are still noticing that you're laying down to sleep during those times, so you're not "wasting" those naps or those days of adaptation.

As long as you start to sleep during your naps within a couple days, and are feeling somewhat better by the end of week one, you should be fine. I've never heard of anyone who started a polyphasic schedule and found that they couldn't sleep at all because of it. (And I had pretty severe insomnia when I started Uberman, remember. I didn't sleep at all until halfway through day two.)

As before, the important thing remains sticking to the schedule:
You lay down on time and you get up on time, no matter what. If you didn't sleep, you may feel crappy, but your brain still noticed that you were laying there and being available for sleep, and that's the important thing. (If you can't sleep, do NOT read, listen to music or "do something else" instead. That time is SLEEP TIME, not to be used for anything else, except perhaps (lying-flat) meditation or relaxation-breathing.)

Remember, it may take several days, or longer, for your brain to click onto the fact that 4:00 PM, a time which has possibly never been a regular sleep-time for you, is now the home of a 20-minute block in which you expect to get restful sleep. It will understand this after you lay down for precisely 20 minutes at 4:00 PM for a while—and that's the *only* way it'll understand.

So don't be upset if you don't fall asleep every time, or if it takes you a long time to fall asleep at first. Just stick to the schedule as doggedly as you can, and your body will catch up with you in a few days.

VI. Adaptation Part Two: Finalizing Adjustment

By the time you get through the first 5–7 days, you should be feeling dramatically better; sleep-dep symptoms should only be happening once or twice a day for short periods of time, and if you keep it up without mistakes, by Day 10 (or earlier) you should feel no deprivation symptoms at all.

The process of adjusting usually works like this: For a day or more, you can't sleep at all, or you only sleep for a nap or two (and then are less than happy when you have to wake up after 20 minutes!). Then you begin to sleep for a nap, or two naps, during the day – that's a good sign that things are progressing. By the end of week one on Uberman, you should be able to sleep for most or all of your scheduled naps, and be only a little tired, if at all, during the night. If you reach day 10 (without major screwups) and you still can't sleep during your naps, and/or you're still feeling terrible at night, something's wrong; you're not adjusting. ...I'd offer advice in that case, but I've yet to see it happen, so I wouldn't stress out about it!

Paying the Price of Everyman

If you're adapting to a core-sleep/non-equiphasic schedule like Everyman, this—the end of week one—is where you pay your debt. Your first few days of adjusting weren't as difficult as those of people adapting to Uberman or Dymaxion, but now they're all done with the hard part, and you're not. There's probably still one, maybe two, times of day that you get really tired, and have to be careful during in order to avoid falling asleep. This is normal, and it's not unusual for it to last several more weeks before you fully adjust. As long as you feel good the rest of the time, and aren't experiencing any symptoms of systemic sleep-deprivation (your memory, coordination, and health are good or improving; and you're sleeping well during at least most of your naps), then you're fine; keep it up and you will adjust. It can be wearying, but Everyman just takes longer—that's its price.

Although you should mostly or entirely stop feeling tired by **the end of week one, the imperative to keep to your schedule exactly remains until at least week three**, preferably four. It's a scientific fact that it takes about a month for the brain to develop a new habit, and that's what you're doing here: Developing the habit of polyphasic sleep. It's a big habit to ingrain, and it doesn't stick easily; so consistency is key. Remember that the habit of sleeping monophasically was ingrained in you, most likely, while you were an infant (and even that probably took several weeks or months of work on your caregiver's part). And you've had the monophasic habit for how many years now? Don't think that breaking it is easy, or that a few days of sleeping differently will do it. Even a month is cutting it close—I suggest at least two months of strict adherence before you risk fudging or modifying your schedule at all, unless you have good reason to believe that something needs changing with your schedule. I'll go over making those changes in the next section, but first:

You Know You're Adapting When...

It's important to know that you ARE adapting, that progress is happening and you're not just making yourself tired for nothing. Especially around the end of the first week, signs of progress are important motivators (extra-especially for Everyman sleepers, who will see slower progress than Uberman-type sleepers). *If you're not sure whether you're making progress in your adaptation, I strongly suggest you start keeping a chart* of your naps. A very simple one will do—you just want to be able to note, for every nap, whether it was on-time, how long you slept, and how you felt before and afterwards.

But whether or not you're keeping formal track, it's good to know that all these are signs that you're adapting to your polyphasic schedule:

During more and more naps, you're able to do one or more of the following:

- Fall asleep quickly

  - Sleep deeply

  - Wake up feeling refreshed

  - You begin to dream during your naps, eventually during at least one nap each day (see the section on "Dreaming" in the next part for more on that)

- You don't yawn or feel tired during the day, except when it's almost time for your nap

- You feel clear-headed and wide awake during most of your waking night-time hours

- You begin to wake up from naps naturally, before your alarm (note: if this never happens, even after you've adjusted, you may need a slightly longer nap)

- Your memory and motor skills are normal[50] (or with Uberman/Dymaxion, sometimes better than normal[51])

...and...

---

50 You may want to test your memory and motor skills before adapting, if you're worried that you might not realize when you're sleep-deprived or if you're adapting. I did this when I was testing the Everyman schedule. I memorized several poems before I took on the schedule, and took typing-tests every day for a week. Then, while I was adjusting, I could take a typing test or see how long it took me to memorize a poem, and know how I was doing. (This is partly why I know that the Everyman adjustment period drags on for a while—it took about 6 weeks for my typing to recover to pre-adaptation levels, even though I felt fine after 3 weeks.)

51 Improvements in cognitive function have been reported from several people who adapted to Uberman/Dymaxion, and were recorded in Stampi's experiment as well. I felt them, too, when I did it, but I did no tests to confirm the effect—others have, though. No, I can't explain what would cause this. Perhaps the nap-only schedules are more efficient in a way that benefits the brain somehow?

You Know You're Having Trouble Adapting When...

After at least one week of perfect[52] adherence to your schedule:

- You regularly have trouble falling asleep; you wake up in the middle of naps; or you wake up exhausted—during more than one nap a day. If you're only having a problem for one specific nap, and another week of strict adherence (2–4 weeks for Everyman) doesn't solve it, then you probably just need tweaking (see next section). But if it's happening for multiple naps every day, then you're not adapting.

- You yawn or feel tired frequently, and not always at the same time(s).

- You feel muddy-headed and stupid all night, or during parts of the day (again, if it's just, or mostly, before or after one particular nap, and doesn't go away on its own, it may be fixable by tweaking).

- You always, or nearly always, feel wiped out and unwilling to wake up when your alarm goes off.

- Your memory and/or motor skills are still markedly, noticeably "off" (note that recovering them fully may take several weeks on Everyman).

Tweaking Your Schedule

"Tweaking" is my term for making a minor adjustment to a polyphasic schedule. Specifically, once you've adjusted, if there's still a "rough spot", you tweak to fix it.

Sometimes, a sleeper gets totally adapted, but still has problems with feeling tired before or after one particular nap, or at a certain time of day, or related to a certain

---

52   Or "amazingly close to perfect"—one ten-minute oversleep doesn't necessarily nullify a whole week, but three hours does.

activity[53]. When this happens, sometimes the schedule needs a "tweak". This may involve moving a nap slightly, or changing the napping environment or other circumstances surrounding your sleep.

Polyphasic sleep is just like regular sleep when it comes to environment and lifestyle. Things like diet, the room you sleep in, and what you do before and after sleeping can have a definite, measurable effect on your sleep. What's more, polyphasic sleep is more efficient, so things that may not have affected your sleep while you were monophasic may have a noticeable effect on your new schedule.

I get a lot of questions about tweaking one's schedule, so let me start with the biggest part of almost all the answers: **About eight times out of ten, if you're having problems adapting, it's not because you need to modify your schedule.** Seven of those eight times, the problem is that you've been trying to cheat your way through the adjustment period—Sleeping extra, skipping or moving naps, using substances to keep yourself awake, or just plain oversleeping. *If that's the case, then attempting to tweak your schedule will just make the problem worse.* There is no easy way to adapt to polyphasic sleep that I know of[54], and more importantly, if there is an easy way, then you—"you" being a generic term for a new polyphaser—probably aren't going to be the one to find it. Don't try polyphasic sleeping unless you intend to go through the adaptation, in all its suck and glory. And if you had a genuine mistake in there that you couldn't avoid, and it threw you off to the point where you're now not adapting properly, then it's time to quit and take a stabilizing break before you try again (see next section).

The other most common reason for adjustment problems is that there's an issue related to behavior or lifestyle that's interfering with your sleep. So before you mess with the schedule you've worked so hard to get (mostly) adapted to, check for things that may be interfering, and address them. (If there's more than one, address them one at a time, leaving at least a few naps between changes.)

---

53   Such as being tired after eating.

54   See Appendix III if you want to read about a possibly-easier adaptation method that I've heard of but can't verify.

With all changes, you should make one, stick with it for long enough that you know it's working (keeping notes if necessary or desired), and then assess whether the change should be kept, expanded upon, or reversed. The first day's effects of a change are not, in my opinion, enough to judge it overall. I like to give my schedule-changes at least two or three days before I call them "keepers" or not.

Keep in mind that what's making you tired may not be directly related to the nap closest to your tiredness: Something making a nap less efficient may be producing tiredness that doesn't show up until a nap or two later. (For me, it's common for a "bad thing" to affect not the nap right after it, but the one after that.) So if you're having problems, look carefully at all your behavior.

Before Tweaking the Schedule: Red-flag Behaviors that are Known to Interfere with Polyphasic Sleep

- **Are you eating too close to a nap?**
  Typically, polyphasers find that eating should be done right after waking up, or in the middle of a waking-cycle; not closer than an hour or two before the time you lay down. Digesting food in the stomach puts you in a deeper sleep and can make you not want to wake up, or wake up sluggishly. If you have digestion issues, they can also interfere with the quality of your sleep.

- **Are you consuming caffeine?**
  Some people are fine with small, controlled amounts of caffeine while sleeping polyphasically; others are not. If you're having problems and you consume caffeine, try limiting and/or changing the time of day that you consume your caffeine, and see if the "problem nap(s)" change in response. If so, you probably need to limit it or cut it out of your diet. (Don't forget that severely limiting caffeine or quitting it can give you a few days' worth of nasty headaches, which may also mess with your sleep. If you can't limit or quit caffeine before becoming polyphasic, then consider doing so slowly, so you don't get the headaches. Gotta love addiction.)

- **Are you consuming alcohol or other drugs (including cigarettes)?**
  Obviously these can affect your sleeping. Try abstaining and see if that fixes

the problem. (If it's something you'll have a withdrawal from, you should probably quit sleeping polyphasically, quit the drug(s), and then try again later.) There's another section on Substances near the end of the book, too.

- **Where and how are you sleeping?**

  - **Do you use a sleep track or sleep to music?**
    If so, maybe you're not getting deep enough sleep due to the noise. If not, maybe you're sleeping too deeply because of the silence. That sounds circular, but for some people, having some noise on (especially at night) keeps them from sinking too far under; while for others it just "inoculates" them to noise and they sleep through their alarms. Being an individual is a b*tch, eh?)

  - **Is your room too warm (which can make it hard to wake up) or too dark (ditto)?**
    We all need our doses of darkness, but if you're sensitive to light and darkness, try getting your dark during the day (i.e. by using a sleep mask) instead of at night. I find that leaving a lamp on during my evening nap (and using a sleep mask) really helps me wake up afterwards. Conversely, if you're too cold or it's too bright, you may not be able to sleep well enough.

  - **Are you sleeping in your bed at night?**
    This can be a bad idea, as your body is trained to "hibernate" in your bed (or wherever you normally sleep at night). At least for a while, try sleeping on the couch, in a recliner, or somewhere else that isn't as comfy and conducive to hours of Z's. Once you're fully adapted, you may find that you can go back to using your bed. (I did.)

- **Are you exercising too close to a nap?**
  This can interfere with the quality of some people's sleep, either by putting them "under" too far (due to exhaustion and the need for muscle repair), or prevent deep sleep due to the body's level of adrenaline and other natural stimulants that are released during exercise. If you're not sleeping well for one or more naps, or having trouble waking up after them, try making sure

you don't exercise strenuously too close beforehand. See the section on Athletics & Exercise later on for more details on this and related issues.

- **Are you mentally too "wound up"?**
  I don't know about you, but I have a terrible time sleeping when my brain is too active. Sometimes, for example when you're expecting to do something scary or exciting right when you wake up, there's not much you can do about having trouble sleeping; but those kinds of incidents should be rare, unless you're such a nervous person that your daily activities freak you out. For other cases, though, such as times of day when you just happen to be very mentally active, there are steps you can take to help yourself wind down and sleep:

  - **Learn deep breathing & relaxation techniques.**
    You can be more in-control of your mind than you think, and one easy way is to learn some deep breathing and/or relaxation techniques. These work immediately, by forcing your mind to stop chewing whatever bone it's gotten ahold of, and encouraging your body to let go of built-up stress—two things that are incredibly helpful for falling asleep.

  - **Get it out physically.**
    If you're really wound up or stressed out and it's nap-time, try exhausting yourself with some fast exercises—pushups and situps work great; so does a punching-bag. Sometimes pent-up stress can be released through physical activity, allowing you to sleep.

  - **Cool down.**
    This works best when one of your naps is just unfortunately scheduled right in the middle of a time you're usually very mentally "awake"—for me, my evening nap (on Everyman) is this way, and it gave me plenty of trouble at first. However, if I make sure to put my feet up and read something either fun and brainless, or technical and boring, for about 15 minutes before that nap, it'll greatly assist me in falling asleep. Other good cool-down activities people have reported to me are having a bath, having a "nightcap" (some kind of small

snack or drink that puts you in a sleeping mood—it certainly doesn't have to be alcoholic), listening to quiet music, or watching scenes from a movie you've seen a hundred times.

- **Learn to meditate**.

  In the interest of full disclosure, I'm a practitioner of Taoism and Chan Buddhism, so it's kind of in my nature to recommend that people learn to meditate. Enlightenment aside, though, meditating regularly can be useful for helping you fall asleep—not just once, but every time; and, I would hazard to say, whether or not you're poly-phasic! Unlike deep breathing/relaxation, meditation is an exercise that conditions you to be more relaxed overall, and more aware of the state of your mind and body. (Meditation often incorporates deep breathing and relaxation, but that's not the point of it—the point, in a nutshell, is to achieve pure awareness, elevated consciousness without thought.) Meditating before sleep can be a nice way to wind down as well, though for some people it actually wakes them up, so try it first and see what works for you[55].

If ~

- You've been sticking to your schedule without mistakes for at least a week (Uberman) or two (Everyman), **and**

- You can tell that you are adapting (see guidelines above), **but**

- There's still a place or two in your 24-hour cycle that you feel tired during almost every day, or a nap you regularly have difficulty falling asleep for, **and**

---

55   I openly recommend that everyone look up information on relaxation and breathing techniques, because those are neutral, proven things, and I don't feel at all weird giving people advice about them. Meditation is another matter, since people have many different ideas of what it is and what it's for, and obviously I have my own ideas, born of my spiritual practice—and I don't want to get preachy about that here. If you'd like to read more of my thoughts on meditation, you can find them on my website (look for the "Better Thinking" category); or if you'd like to discuss it with me, feel free to drop me a line.

- You've already tried modifying all the behaviors which may be causing the interference,

Then (and only then!)

You should consider "Tweaking" your schedule.

The Tweaking Process

Tweaking a schedule is like (very like, heh) troubleshooting a mechanical or computer problem: You pick one small change that looks likely, make it, and watch for a while. If the problem is unaffected, or gets worse, you "back off" the change, making it smaller or eliminating it entirely. If things get better, but not enough, you "turn up" the change, adding a little to it and then watching, adding, watching, until you're satisfied with the result. If one change doesn't work, you pick another one and start over.

In this case, the "changes" you're making are changes in your nap-times or dura-tions. Again, Nap Tweaking should be a last resort—it's so much easier to diagnose and fix behavioral problems, and much more likely that that will fix your issue. So we're assuming here that you've already tried fixing all the likely behavioral issues, diet issues, sleep circumstances, etc. outlined above; and it still hasn't worked. But it is true that, for people on Everyman schedules especially, Tweaking is sometimes necessary in order to get things down smooth. Tweaking an equiphasic (Uberman or Ubermanlike[56]) schedule is more difficult, and more likely to cause problems, so be extra careful if this is what you're doing.

In all cases, be minimalist, though—polyphasic schedules require more regularity and consistency than an average 8-hour monophasic schedule does, so don't think that just because you can move your waking or sleeping-times a lot while you're monophasic, that will still be necessarily true when you're polyphasic.

---

56 Would this be written "Ubermanly"?? Gods, I hope not!

If you have to Tweak, here are good places to start. Remember to make one change, and to wait at least a few days to see if it should be kept, kept and built upon, backed off a bit, or reversed, before making another change. Also, consider writing down how you feel immediately before or after sleeping, for some or all of you naps. Small changes to your sleep can be especially hard to keep track of if you don't write things down.

Tweaks to Try:

- **If you are regularly tired after waking from a certain nap** (and have addressed possible behavioral reasons), and you're usually tired before this nap, move it 15 minutes closer to the one before it. If this helps a little but not enough, move it another 15 minutes, and so forth.

- **If you regularly have trouble falling asleep for a certain nap** (and have addressed possible behavioral reasons), and are usually not tired right before this nap, move the nap 15 minutes farther away from the one before it. Remember, this might work "too well", leaving you waking up groggy—if that happens, back it off and try just 7 minutes instead of fifteen. Changes that small do make a difference sometimes.

- If you have trouble falling asleep and are tired right before your nap, consider shortening the duration of all your naps by 2–5 minutes, especially if they're currently longer than 20 minutes total[57]. Some people do better with naps that are 18 or even 15 minutes long. This fix can also help if you're always groggy immediately upon waking up from some or all of your naps.

    - There's a tendency to want to lengthen your naps if you feel you aren't getting enough rest—counterintuitively, this rarely helps. If you're waking up groggy, the most likely reason is that you've slept too hard

---

57 Although Dr. Fuller proscribed 30-minute naps for his "Dymaxion" schedule, in my experience and those of the many people I've spoken to, in the ballpark of 20 minutes always seems to work better. I would even go so far as to say that maybe Dr. Fuller was estimating ("about half an hour"), or that he was simply not the norm.

or too long, so that instead of waking up neatly at the end of a "cycle" of sleep (which cycles happen about every 20 minutes during a nap), you've entered the beginning of the next cycle, and are interrupting it when you wake. So try shortening a nap before lengthening one, unless you're already at or below the 15-minute mark (though I did speak with someone whose comfortable nap-duration was 13 minutes, so that is possible too).

- As you adapt, your nap-duration may naturally shorten; don't let this worry you. If you're adapted and you wake up just a few minutes before your alarm, feeling refreshed, you can get up; if this happens regularly, you may want to set your alarms a little earlier, so that they catch you at the "right time".

- **If you're on Everyman and always tired after waking up from your core nap** (and have addressed behavioral issues, which are very common surrounding a core nap), try taking it half an hour earlier. If you naturally have low energy at night, you may be pushing your waking-period too far and getting overtired.

    - If that doesn't work, try shortening your core by 15 minutes, then half an hour. If the problem persists, try lengthening it by 15 minutes. The 1.5, 3, and 4.5-hour suggested durations of core naps are based on a 90-minute sleep cycle, which is normal but not universal—yours may be a little different. Sometimes even 5 or 10 minutes' duration of a core nap can mean the difference between waking tired and waking up refreshed. Pay attention to your body—if subtracting 15 minutes helps but not very much, try 20.

- **Don't be afraid to try other changes if you feel you need to. Just remember**—make them one at a time, and keep them small, and give a few days to each to see how it affects you. For some people, finding just the right schedule takes months of "detective work", but keep in mind that you're not tired during that whole month; just a little sleepy before or after a certain nap or during a certain time of day. For many people (including me), that still represents an improvement over how they felt on a monophasic schedule. And don't give up—once you're adapted, you know you can sleep polyphasically, and it's just a matter of sanding off the rough edges. Your "perfect" schedule may take a little discovering, but it's there.

As you can see, getting a schedule just right means tailoring it to your particular sleep cycle, so that you're waking up when you've finished one "cycle" and before you begin another one.

A note on sleep cycles: There are several ways to "measure" your sleep cycles, including going to a sleep lab, buying a device (or even, as of recently, an app for your phone) that will measure it, or even just having someone who knows what to look for watch you sleep and take notes. However, this is of limited usefulness if you do it before you adapt to polyphasic sleep, because adapting to the new schedule will probably change how your sleep-cycles work, at least a little.

If you really want to get a "technical" knowledge of your sleep cycles and how they work, though, those tools can be quite handy; go ahead and use them. Knowledge hardly ever hurts, when it comes to sleeping better!

Such technical knowledge isn't necessary, though, even for Tweaking—most people are surprised to find out how easily they can "feel" when they've woken in the beginning, middle or end of a sleep-cycle. Since the 20-minute nap works well, as a base, for almost everybody, you should know what "waking up rested and in-between cycles" feels like, by the time you get to the point of Tweaking. After that, it's just a matter of testing different configurations and seeing which ones get you closest to feeling rested from that particular nap.

Figuring out where your sleep-cycles are and what lengths of naps work and don't can sound like a daunting task, but keep in mind that while you're doing all that experimenting, you're still adapted and probably feeling mostly great. For many people, being tired before or after a nap or two is quite a lot less tiredness than they experienced while being monophasic! So don't interpret "you may spend months tweaking to get this just right" to mean that you'll be miserable and tired for months—you may be fine; and in fact many people decide to just deal with one nap being a little hard to wake up from or go down for, without bothering to tweak at all. As far as I know, there's nothing harmful about taking that road either.

If Tweaking Doesn't Work

Sometimes, for some reason, even tweaking a schedule won't produce a situation where you're never tired. You may find that it's always a struggle to wake from your core or a certain nap, or that you always get a bit yawny around 3 AM no matter what you do.

There are two things you should do in this situation. The first is to **assess your health**: How do you feel? Are you feeling any worse as you continue to sleep polyphasically? While in my experience polyphasic sleep can work for almost anybody who can physically and mentally handle the adjustment, it *is* a more efficient method of sleeping, and it's reasonable to assume that not everyone has the constitution to increase the efficiency of an involuntary physical processes as complex as sleeping[58].

If your health is okay, though, and you don't feel (or have evidence that) polyphasic sleep is doing any damage to you, then it's time to ask another question: **How do you feel compared to when you were monophasic?** Are you tired more or less of the time? Do you have more or less energy, and how is your stress level? If things are better for you being polyphasic, it may be worth it to deal with the occasional tiredness for however many months it takes you to figure out what will eliminate it. But if you generally don't feel as good, then maybe you're just a monophasic sleeper.

The trick, then, is to know when to quit trying to adapt.

When To Give Up

There's a danger limit, which I've tried to mention regularly throughout this book; a limit to how much you can mess with a central biological process like sleep and not suffer any consequences—and by "consequences" I mean:

---

58   Most people without the constitution for polyphasic sleeping simply don't want to do it, in my experience—they know, on some level, that they need and prefer longer, "slower" sleep. But it is possible that psychologically, you could desire to sleep polyphasically, but not be meant for it physically.

- Making yourself ill;

- Hurting your performance for so long that your life suffers; or

- "Ruining" your sleep schedule, by training yourself not to be monophasic, but not replacing that with any other fixed schedule.

Those are, as far as I'm aware, the worst outcomes of a failed attempt at adapting to polyphasic sleep. All of them are caused when irregular, non-scheduled sleeping goes on for too long, which means that it's important, if you're not succeeding at adapting to a polyphasic schedule, that you recognize this and stop trying before you face icky consequences. Unfortunately, due to the nature of sleep deprivation, it can be difficult to know when you're near that limit.

Therefore, it's extremely important to keep an eye on your progress, and to know when you need to quit, at least for a while. (I've said this already, but if you can find a sympathetic friend who understands what you're doing and won't jump the gun, it can be helpful to give them the power—as your "kill switch"—to make you call it quits.)

Generally speaking, if you've been trying to sleep polyphasically for a month or more, and you can't keep to a regular schedule, then it's time to quit. Whether you feel it or not, you're sleep-deprived from all the irregular sleep, and if you sleep irregularly for any longer, you risk training your mind and body to not sleep on a schedule at all. This can ruin your chances for a good night's sleep entirely, and even land you on medication or under medical care before your schedule can recover. So don't push it! If you didn't succeed at adapting this time, take a long break, take some notes, make careful preparations, and try again later.

Needless to say, you should also quit if you experience any really adverse effects, such as dramatic weight gain or loss, illness, or psychological meltdown. Those would be, you know, bad.

When you "quit", make sure it's for at least 30 days (60 is even better), and that you re-establish a regular monophasic or biphasic schedule for that whole time. It's really important to give enough time in there that you can re-establish some regular sleep-schedule, and also to get enough rest to make up for any sleep-deprivation that may have "built up" (yes, it builds up) while you were trying to adapt.

While you're at it, too, why not make some observations about your "normal" sleep habits, with an eye to things that may have sabotaged your polyphasic attempt? A period of rest or quitting can be an ideal time to:

- quit caffeine or other stimulants or drugs

- improve your sleep environment

- establish good sleep habits

- modify your diet or exercise routine

- accustom yourself to living on a schedule, if you're not already used to it

Sometimes the second time is the charm, especially if you've learned from the first time and use the break to prepare. (The first time I adapted, I did it in one shot—which is good, because I might not have tried again!—but the next time, it took me two tries. My lifestyle was very different, and I didn't expect the problems I would have... but when I tried again, knowing what to expect, it worked.) So be smart about quitting when you should quit, and don't worry that it necessarily means giving up for good!

VII. Living Polyphasically

This section is devoted to issues that primarily concern polyphasic sleep as a lifestyle—which, in my own personal definition, means "as done for more than four months consecutively". I pick four months because there seems to be a certain "swing of things" that kicks in after five or six months, so it seemed as good a place as any to distinguish long-term from short-term polyphasic schedules.

That's not to say that short-term polyphasic sleep isn't useful, or that everyone who adapts to a polyphasic schedule does or should do so with the aim of staying on it for years. But many people, once they get through the "Hell week" part of it, find that they like polyphasic sleep a lot, and keep to the schedule as long as they can. Sometimes life interferes, but the good news is, once you've adapted successfully to a polyphasic schedule once, it seems to be easier to do it again. Someone in a polyphasic-related forum once theorized that maybe there's a "nap switch" in your brain, and once you flip that switch—once you learn to nap, and to use naps as an efficient replacement for nighttime sleep—then you never really forget how. It was certainly easier for me to adapt to my schedule the second time around (once the lifestyle issues were resolved); I got the hang of falling asleep and waking rested much more quickly than I thought I would.

Polyphasic sleep in the long-term seems to be a much different animal than it is while you're adapting, and also somewhat different than it is for the first 6 months or so after adaptation. I'll address some of the things that have seemed notable, difficult or relevant to me as I've slept polyphasically over the last three years; however, everyone is invited to remember that I'm one of relatively few[59] people doing this at the moment, and there's no long-term study data at all on polyphasic sleep at the moment.

---

59   It used to be "very few", but as of the Second Edition, this is no longer true—I've actually lost count of other long-term polyphasers now!

The Changing Nature of Screwing Up

Do you know anyone who goes to bed at precisely, say, 10:42 every night, and wakes at exactly 5:23? Every single day? Me neither. Polyphasic schedules are super-strict by necessity while you're adapting to them, and even after that, they remain stricter than monophasic schedules, because they're more stripped-down and efficient. But it's not Perfectly Strict For All Time. And once you've really, truly got the hang of it, "screw-ups" that would have completely nuked your schedule in the past become quite easy to work around, and it all just blends together into a full-grown specimen of sleep schedule. A weird specimen to be sure, but on many levels just like any other.

Here's an example: If I miss a nap, or move one too far out of its usual position in the day, I will start to get tired about 11 PM. Always happens. If I stay up until 1 a.m. anyway, I will be quite resistant to waking up in the morning, and maybe also be a little sleepy after my morning nap; but if I go to bed early, at 11:30, I'll be fine at 4 AM. In short, if I sleep 4.5 hours instead of 3, I can recover almost totally from having missed a nap (though I still feel a bit sluggish from oversleeping at first). If I just push through it and sleep the normal three hours, I'll recover as well, but only after experiencing some morning tiredness. Generally I pick which thing I want to do to recover from a missed nap depending on how I feel that day, how much I have to do, etc.

Another example: If I have to do something that will make me miss a nap or move it too far, and I know about it ahead of time, I may take a 10 or 15-minute nap before-hand. That'll keep me from being too tired, and I'll take my normal nap when I can, if I can. Depending on how that shakes out, I might be tired when I wake up from the next nap...

In other words, life on a polyphasic schedule is a steady dance of trying to keep your sleep-schedule on track so that you're not tired, and mitigating the tiredness when you can't avoid messing with your schedule. That may sound odd, but if you stated how a normal (monophasic) sleep schedule works, it would sound almost exactly the same. A monophaser might say, "If I'm stressed-out and can't get to sleep right away, then I'm going to be pretty wasted in the morning. If I can, I'll sleep in by 2 hours and that will help, but if I can't sleep in and I can't get a nap tomorrow afternoon, I'm going to be yawning all day." The numbers are smaller with polyphasic sleep, but the principle – and it seems, at least in general, the ratios – are the same.

Real life makes you modify your schedule on-the-fly sometimes; it just does. Polyphasic sleep is no different, once it's in full swing. The difference is the work it takes to get to "full swing"[60].

And being fully adapted isn't an on/off thing either: For a while, you're going to have to use your brain to decide when to sleep and when not to, because your habits are still going to lead to you to want to sleep at night, even if you don't need to. After long enough, though, it becomes a "gut decision"; napping becomes your normal schedule, and you no longer tend to sleep all night, even if you want to (or try!).

I watch the clock much less now: When it's nearing bedtime I get tired, and for most of my naps I wake up automatically at the right time. For those naps that I tend to oversleep (because they happen at low-energy parts of my day, or because I'm likely to have had to move the nap prior), I use alarms and a cattleprod incentives to get myself up. ☺ The best incentives remain those that are interesting: I'll start a project, prep some food to cook, or watch the first 15 minutes of a movie before I lay down, and then getting going again is usually a snap. Of course, I could just as easily have taken those steps to mitigate morning tiredness on my monophasic schedule, but **one of the virtues of polyphase for me has definitely been that it makes me pay closer attention**. I think it does this for a lot of people, and while that's awesome on a level, it's also problematic, because without real scientific study, it's hard to separate how much of the benefit of polyphasic sleep is the schedule itself, and how much is paying closer attention to how you sleep and how you feel!

---

60   To be fair, this may not be different at all. Anyone who's trained a baby to sleep at night can tell you that consistency helps a lot there, too; and that it's often not an easy adjustment!

On my blog, I talk very little about which naps I got or missed, and how I compensated for them[61]. This is simply because it gets tiring, constantly saying, "THIS INFORMATION ONLY APPLIES IF YOU'RE MORE THAN SIX MONTHS IN." ...Most of my readers aren't. And even if I issue that disclaimer, it hardly ever works, and I end up getting a bunch of questions from people who want to make those kinds of modifications early on. (I don't mean to sound ungrateful—I enjoy the questions I get, for the most part.) Almost nobody who reads my website is a long-term polyphasic sleeper (there are a few; but what do they need my advice for anyway?), and I felt that I was confusing too many of the readers I have who are trying to adapt[62]. For people who are adapting (on any level), a screwup is a screwup—it will make them sleep-deprived and delay, or ruin, their success at living on a polyphasic schedule. For the completely adapted, a (minor) screwup is just a blip on the radar that gets fixed later. Big lifestyle events and changes that would ruin a normal monophasic schedule will ruin your polyphasic one too; but once you're completely adapted, having to re-adapt (after illness, travel, or what have you) isn't much harder than getting back on a monophasic schedule is—the only thing that makes it hard, then, is the world's tendency to expect you to be asleep at night!

In other words, adaptation is hardcore. After that, once you're used to the schedule, things get a bit squishier and it starts feeling and acting like a "regular" sleep/wake pattern. But getting used to the schedule brings its own challenges, too...

Getting Bored

Besides the change in the nature of screwups, something else that tends to happen long-term is that boredom becomes a problem. Everyone I've spoken to who did long-term polyphase talked about, at one point or another, having to deal with being up at night and being boooorrrred and really wanting to just go to sleep and fast-forward some time.

---

61   This is less true in recent years; I'm now more of a long-term polyphaser than anything, and and long-term polyphasic sleep is more common now, so I talk about it more often.

62   Plus—I won't hide it—I hate repeating myself. Pet peeve.

I'm sure this doesn't happen to everyone. I bet Einstein could have stayed awake for days and days and not gotten bored, but most of us aren't lucky enough to have a brain that fascinating, and for even very industrious folk, living on a 20+-hour day is likely to get wearisome at times. There's also a psychological component that shouldn't be ignored: Your mind can only handle so much stimulation, and sometimes that feeling that you just don't wanna do anything is directly related to the fact that, mentally and/or emotionally, you've hit a limit to the experiences you can absorb for a while. I'm sure those limits, too, are different for everyone.

Needless to say, if the boredom is endemic or systemic, then you've got a bigger problem with being polyphasic—but it feels safe to assume that, if you were bored all the time, you wouldn't have reached the point of total adaptation, which is what we're discussing here. So we'll assume from here on that you may experience boredom, but only occasionally. In which case, you have a few options for how to handle it. Some of these ideas seem contradictory, but that's because different things work for different people... start with an educated guess and if that doesn't work, try something else.

- **Follow a schedule**.
  Sometimes you just get sick of *thinking of the next thing to do* - I know I do. Building a schedule, either for your entire day or just for the times you tend to get bored, can be an easy way out in that case.

- **Pick a "default activity"**.
  This is a great, if somewhat obvious, idea if you're the type who loves to do a certain thing, or is in the middle of a big project: Make yourself devote any time that isn't already devoted to something else, to that thing. You'll get more done, and if you get sick of it for a while, it'll be incentive not to let yourself get bored. A win-win situation, really.

- **Whip out the icky stuff**.
  Make a list of useful things you hate doing: laundry, bills, some irritating personal care requirement, or whatever. Label it "Bored List" or something more creative if you like, and do something off it whenever you get bored. If you're the right kind of personality, then having the list out there, looming with its Ick, will keep you from letting yourself get bored. And if you do

get bored, well, at least something useful gets done. If you're not the right kind of personality, though, the presence of this list can lead you to doing not-good things, or oversleeping, in order to avoid having to pull out the list. (The list, in this case, is similar to my mom, who would give you chores if you complained of boredom. If moms like mine could motivate you, this probably will too.)

- **Go low-key once in a while**.
  If your problem is mental or emotional exhaustion[63], you may find yourself getting "bored", or entering a state where nothing you could do sounds palatable, even if you have lots of options and willpower. Sometimes the best thing is to stop trying to accomplish something, and put yourself in standby for a while. I like to read, with no music or computer or other electronic noise anywhere near me. Other people are happy watching a fish-tank, or walking aimlessly, or watching a movie. People need those things occasionally, and a lot of polyphasers get so involved in being hyper-efficient with their time that they forget to just chill once in a while. Make sure you don't waste too much time, though: set a timer or alarm, so your chill-out period is what you need and not too much more.

- **Go ahead and sleep[64]**.
  Obviously, be *extremely careful* with this one, since you risk doing damage to that schedule you worked so hard on, and ending up with a bunch of tiredness to deal with later! Remember that on a polyphasic schedule, more sleep isn't necessarily more refreshing, so try to get away from thinking that "extra" sleep will somehow make you feel better later[65]. Unless you're very

---

63 A good way to determine this is to look at what you've been doing all day—if it's very brain-intensive, or difficult emotionally (i.e. if you're a professor or a therapist, etc.) then it's likely that that part of you is tiring out, even though your body isn't. You see this a lot in students, even monophasic ones, who are working a really intensive program: After doing it most of the day, they tend to shut down, and either stare at walls or get drunk.

64 My gods, did I just say that?? ☺

65 The obvious exception being if you're sick, in which case you DO need extra sleep. See next section for more on that.

careful, and possibly even if you are, extra sleep will actually make you feel more tired, or at least you'll have some trouble waking up at some point. However, if you know your schedule and yourself well, you've probably figured out some place where you can fit some extra Zs if you want to, and not suffer for it. Even Uberman schedules seem to have those places, once they're done long enough. I suggest making a list of when it is and isn't acceptable to get any extra sleep (include times of day, durations, and things you want to definitely have accomplished first—you'll be shocked how much time you lose to sleep, if you're used to polyphasic naps), so that you're not making the decision when you're bored and *want* to sleep. Also, make sure you don't use this option too often—once a week should be the maximum, really. "Loosening up" your schedule too much can lead to an erratic schedule and systemic tiredness—it's less of a danger for adapted polyphasers, but you can't just give up on your schedule and do whatever, either.

Scheduling Around Real Life

Ah, real life... it could almost be defined as "the stuff that gets in the way of your plans", couldn't it? Long-term polyphasers seem to run the gamut between carefully scheduling all their time, and scheduling little more than their naps. I'm probably a 7 out of 10 on the scheduling scale—I have a proposed schedule for each day, that I modify as needed on an ongoing basis. But it doesn't matter how precise you are with your schedule, because nothing can stop Real Life from throwing its monkeywrenches in. The question is, when it does, how does a polyphaser handle them?

Sickness

Almost everyone gets sick sometimes. If you get sick terribly often or badly, you probably don't want to mess with polyphasic sleep anyway; but if you're a normal, healthy person, you probably still deal with colds or allergies or what have you. (Though I'm not saying they're inevitable... I think many regular illnesses are caused by lifestyle. My website has lots of information on typical-illness home remedies and preventions, if that's something that interests you.) And there are things like the flu, food poisoning, and other contagions that sometimes you just get stuck with.

Sickness is the one instance where I've never advocated trying to keep to one's schedule—be it polyphasic or monophasic or whatever. Sickness is not something to mess around with, and it's well-known scientifically that sleep provides some of the best chance for your body to heal. It lets you shut down all non-essential functions and re-route the engines to life support, if you will. ☺ And it's WAY healthier than taking drugs! So whatever your normal sleep schedule, if you've contracted some illness, forget about it—sleep as often as you want and as long as your body will. Feel no shame about staying in bed all day if that's what feels right. I'm all about efficiency, right? Well, missing one day of work to sleep off an illness is way more efficient than missing four to ten days because you wore yourself down to a stub and got hammered with some cold or flu or something!

Many people worry about getting their polyphasic schedule back after a period of illness. This makes sense, especially since our societies tend to be monophasic, so it's naturally easier to fall back into a monophasic rather than a polyphasic schedule. **The most important thing I know of to ensure that you get your schedule back with minimal adjustment and discomfort is to take naps on time, always**. If I sleep from midnight to 8 AM while sick, and wake up feeling energetic, I'll get up and then go back to bed an hour later for my 9 AM nap. I might not be able to sleep, but I lay down anyway, and set my alarm, and get up when it goes off. Any time I'm awake while it's "naptime", I lay down for my 20 minutes. As long as I do that, getting back on-schedule is easy.

One thing that's different when you're sick, or getting sick, is that you probably will crash; rather than sleeping three or four hours, you probably will sleep seven or eight. That is, in fact, one of the key ways that I've learned to tell that I *am* fighting off an illness—if I'm just feeling crappy and I go to bed, I'll sleep three, four and a half, or maybe even six hours... but I won't sleep eight unless there's actually something physical going on. (Which I usually then will wake up without a trace of, because eight hours of sleep is the best medicine.)

I even think it makes sense to sleep extra if you think you *might* be getting sick, provided you can tell. Some people don't notice illness until there are actual symptoms of it—if that's true for you, then you have no way to benefit from a judicious long-nap-to-head-off-illness, and attempting one will probably only fudge up your schedule. Personally though, I can feel when my immune system is strained or engaged in a heated battle. I usually get flushed in the face, my joints become sore, eyes are dry, and I often get vertigo. This happens when I work way longer than normal, when I've been around people who are sick, or when I've been through something especially emotionally taxing. If I keep plowing through that feeling, I'm very likely to come down with something. BUT if I take an extra nap or two, or sleep in for a long core, I can almost always return things to normal. (If I get a bit of a sore throat, that's my red flag—I'm *definitely* going to get ill. When that happens, I take a ton of vitamins and sleep eight hours, stat. As long as I do this on the very first day I notice the sore throat, it usually works!)

Sleep is an amazingly effective remedy: I've found that if I can stay mostly in bed for one or two days, I can "kick" almost any illness I've got, usually with no more medication than lots of water and herbal tea. But this seems to work even better on a polyphasic schedule! One awesome thing that seems to be true about polyphasic sleep is that LESS SLEEP DOES MORE to restore your body and mind to a healthy state. On a monophasic schedule, I used to sleep 8–10 hours to help "fight something off", and 12 or more if I was truly sick. Over the years I've been sleeping polyphasically, those numbers have dropped to 4–6 hours for an effective immune-system boost, and almost never more than 8 hours consecutively. Four hours' sleep feels like a full night to me; six hours feels like sleeping way in; and eight feels like hibernating[66]! Your results may vary of course, but it makes sense to me that once you get used to sleeping only as much as you need (i.e. on a very efficient schedule like a polyphasic one), then sleeping a little extra goes a long way.

The general rule that I espouse for periods of illness and near-illness is this: Your body needs sleep to heal. Give it! Keep taking your naps to stay in the habit, and worry about re-adjusting to less sleep after you're healthy. **Re-adjusting after illness is usually painless if you're already fully adapted**: one day of extra sleep to combat illness does nothing to me; more than one day, and I'll be tired for a night,

---

66   Eight also has a detriment: If I sleep this long, my back will be sore when I wake up. Ick!

two at maximum, while I re-adjust. But it's nothing an interesting phone conversation or a good movie can't combat.

Lastly, even though this section concerns schedules that are already firmly in place, I will mention this: If you're still adjusting, sickness will throw you off completely. Rather than sleep for one or two days and then try to jump right back into your adjustment, I suggest taking a full-stop break for at least a week. There are two reasons for this: One, you want to make sure you're *completely* healthy before you try again. And two, if you slept a whole day during your adaptation, your adaptation is pretty much over, so you need to re-stabilize your sleep before trying again anyway.

Travel

It can be very hard to nap while traveling. Sometimes being able to sleep for short periods and then be rested, and also being able to sleep in strange places, are very valuable skills for the traveler. But for me, the combination of strange places, different food, new things to do, stress, jet-lag, and the necessary nap-shifting that airports and activities can cause, throws my schedule right off. I try to nap while I'm traveling, but mostly I just thank goodness that I don't travel more often, and prepare to have to re-adjust when I return. Re-adjusting gets easier the longer I'm on this schedule, too.

I should note that, though my schedule almost always gets mangled when I travel, I don't generally go back to being monophasic. I make an effort to stay awake during my waking-hours and sleep, or at least lay down, during the times that are supposed to be my naps. As a result, my schedule may get erratic and I may be occasionally tired, but I can slide back into my polyphasic schedule when the trip is over-with. On the other hand, I have been on at least one extended trip when the hosts are filling every day with non-nap-friendly activities, and then being stuck in someone else's house at night with not much to do... and then I have gone monophasic for those few days. Thankfully I had already been polyphasic for over a year when this first happened, and getting back on schedule once I got home wasn't hard – it took less than a week to get right back in the swing of things. Still, my advice is to keep up as much of your schedule as possible while you're traveling, as this will make getting back on track easier when you get home.

It seems that the esteemed Buckminster Fuller was pretty good at napping while traveling[67], and on top of that there are more nap-friendly destinations in the world these days. In very modern places like Tokyo, napping is becoming more and more mainstream, and a place to crash for 20 minutes is relatively easy to find.

I don't travel too much, but over the years now I've done it enough to put together this **list of travel items** it helps, as a polyphasic traveler, to keep close at hand:

- An eye-pillow or blindfold of some sort

- A small timer you can use *that is not attached to your cell-phone* (since you may want to shut off and/or hide your phone while you nap)

- A small blanket—not only to cover yourself, but so that you can put items in your lap and cover them

- Earplugs and/or headphones (again, it helps to have an mp3 player that is not your cellphone, if you want music)—note that in public places[68], you may want to reconsider headphones, since they do kind of scream, "Look over here, I'm sleeping and there are electronics to steal!"

- Water (which you should kind of have while traveling anyway), and small hard candies/cough drops in case your throat is dry or itchy

- An extra jacket or sweater, either for wearing or for rolling up as a pillow

- A sign you can hold, or pen and paper to make a sign. In some places, like airports, you don't have to announce that you're sleeping, since people do it all the time. But if you're crashing somewhere with no napping accom-

---

67   At least, he traveled a good amount and was polyphasic for two years, so one assumes he was. Also, there is a brief anecdote about him being able to pass out on a plane for 30 minutes and wake up refreshed. For my part, I find plane-rides much more aggravating since I've become polyphasic, since I know I can't sleep through the boring part of the trip. On my list: Get a pilot's license!

68   See "Sleeping in Public" near the end of the book for more such tips.

modations and you decide to make do with the car parked outside, it can be incredibly useful to have a sign in your lap that says something like "Napping, please leave me alone; I'll wake up in a few minutes". I've had people bang on the window of a car, or even shake me, because they were worried that I was passed out or injured!

- Small packable hammock/sleeping bag, if you have one

Emergencies

Life is never without emergencies for very long. Being polyphasic can come in very handy in the occasional emergency; or at least, it can be as useful as it is annoying. Needing to sleep every couple hours can be irritating if there's heavy stuff going on; on the other hand, being able to stay awake almost all the time can be a lifesaver. Sometimes, emergencies completely whack your schedule, by making it impossible to get naps, or impossible to sleep due to stress. Other times, they turn out to be perfect times to be polyphasic...

Emergency Uberman

If you can safely and regularly get your daytime naps, then transitioning into Uberman (from any variety of Everyman) is possible and relatively easy, and it can be a wonderful tool for really difficult times. Nothing beats those 20-minute naps for helping you sit up all night with a sick kid, or man a hospital waiting-room, or attend a very late emergency meeting, etc.

I've found that doing Uberman for one or two days (I've never had to do it longer, except when it was my regular schedule) is pretty easy[69] under emergency conditions, and it lets me effectively "not sleep" for as long as I have to. There's no crash afterwards, either, unless it's emotional. (eek.)

---

69 The exhaustion of not getting your core nap makes sleeping for the 20-minute naps pretty easy right off the bat, and the emergency conditions make waking up from those naps almost effortless.

Uberman is also, I've discovered, an amazing tool for long road-trips. Four hours is usually great timing for filling up the tank and emptying the bladder, and grabbing a 20-minute nap at the same time allows for nearly unlimited continuous drive-time. I've done this several times with fifteen-hour trips, and it's been brilliant.

To switch from Everyman to Emergency Uberman, simply skip your core(s) and take 20-minute naps every four hours, with as little variation as you can manage. If you're already on Uberman, obviously you'll want to get your naps if at all possible, since they mean the difference between being alert and fine (no matter how long you go without a night's sleep!) and being a bit of a zombie. If you've adapted to Uberman, though, you're probably used to telling the world to scram for a few minutes while you nap—you just may have to say it more forcefully if the crap is hitting the fan in some way.

Probably the best thing to say about emergencies is to remember that one of the undisputed, frequent uses of polyphasic sleep is by the military, in situations where soldiers are stuck behind enemy lines for long periods of time and can't afford to sleep for hours. Don't feel guilty about drawing a parallel between that and doing time in the hospital waiting-room: Some may stare, but most people would be impressed with your fortitude if they knew you were napping so that you could stay awake near-continuously for days (even months!) on end if you had to.

If you like to be prepared, then don't forget to include a timer (and eye-mask, if you use one) in your emergency kit! (I keep some in my car.)

Re-Adjusting

If you were fully adapted and you kept taking your naps whenever possible, re-adjusting after an illness, vacation, emergency, or similar "real life intrusion" is actually, in my experience, very easy. Simply pick your old schedule (sleep-schedule and daily schedule, if you have one) back up as soon as you can. If you're worried about tiredness, take the same steps you took for your first adjustment—i.e., make another Big Fat List of things to keep yourself occupied with; get some extra alarms; etc. You probably will not need them for very long. In my experience, usually in 1–3 days, you're right back to being fully adapted, and the transition is never as bad as it was when you first adapted—or hasn't been for me, anyway, and I've lost track of how many times I've readjusted due to travel, emergency, or other SNAFU. The only time you need to avoid those things is during adaptation; the rest of the time, it's just a matter of convenience.

In the years since the First Edition, I've also deliberately dropped my polyphasic schedule for a few months and tried to go back to "regular" sleeping, as well as experienced plenty more inconveniences that knocked me off-schedule for a few days or weeks at a time. Each time I had to re-adapt, though, it was easier. I'm now to the point where the last two times I had to re-adapt after being knocked off my schedule (even if I was off-schedule for several weeks), it's been almost painless, with maybe one night of feeling tired, and a few daytime naps I couldn't sleep for.

This fits with what we know about habit-forming in general: Things you do over and over for years are easier to slide back into, even after a long break. Think of the phrase "you never forget how to ride a bicycle". Maybe I will never forget how to nap? (That would be awesome!!)

Missing Sleep

Counterintuitively, polyphasic sleep seems to me to be more flexible than mono-phasic when it comes to re-adjusting.

A monophasic person can miss a whole night's sleep, or get broken sleep, and feel like poop, but usually be functional—once. If they have to do it for another day, or more, things deteriorate rapidly, and it takes ⅓ to ½ of a *day* for them to sleep enough to recover.

But broken sleep for me is much easier to fix: If I miss a nap, or get rudely woken up before one is finished, all I need is an extra nap at some point, or even just a full day of getting all my naps as planned, and I won't even notice. Even if I miss a nap (including my core) completely, if I can fit an extra nap in at all, I will recover, significantly if not entirely, just from that 20 minutes of sleep. If I can get two or three naps at a proper interval, I can erase a whole day's worth of missed naps and broken cores (see the bit on "Emergencies", which is usually when this happens).

For most polyphasers, all that's needed to restore lost sleep is to catch an extra nap, or an hour and a half core. If that's not possible, a few days of sticking to the schedule will generally do it too.

And what's more, I can't speak for others, but personally I can maintain that—missing naps or losing sleep and replacing them with extra naps when I can—for many days without suffering too badly in terms of performance or health.

Some people argue that a polyphasic schedule is easier to mess up than a mono-phasic one, since it requires successfully sleeping 4–6 times a day, instead of once. A valid counter-argument is that monophasers have to stay successfully asleep for a third of a day without interruption in order to be rested, whereas a polyphaser only needs less than half an hour of uninterrupted sleep at a time! And as described above, a polyphasic schedule is also, in my opinion, a lot easier to fix. Naps may come annoyingly often and be aggravatingly difficult to catch during an emergency or other shakeup; but it takes much less sleep, overall, to recover a polyphasic schedule from "Real Life" intrusions.

Eating & Substances

I get a lot of questions about diet and medicines, and I wish I knew the answers to more of them, or that I could provide more foundation for the answers I do know than, "This is what happened to me," or "This is what others have told me." (To be fair, I can also use "My mom is a nurse" and "I make herbal medicines in my kitchen sometimes", but nobody seems really impressed by those either.) But this is what I know, and what I've learned, that could be useful:

- **Can I eat anything I want, when I want?**
  It's nothing new that eating affects your sleep, but as with most things, the consequences are more noticeable on a polyphasic schedule. Some effects are easy to spot: You shouldn't eat a lot too close before a nap, because you'll sleep either too hard or not well, depending on your body's digestion process. You should be careful with foods that are stimulants, like caffeine and sugar; use them sparingly and with an eye to your sleep-times. You may also want to stay away from turkey, warm milk and other foods that might

make you tired, during adaptation or a time of day you're likely to over-sleep. ...Other than those things, I'm not aware of any specific restrictions being polyphasic imposes. If you feel that you might have problems being polyphasic because of the times, amounts, or types of food that you need to eat, you may want to discuss it with one of the groups of polyphasic sleepers on the Internet, who are often chock-full of advice and suggestions. (See the Resources section.)

- **Can I be vegan/vegetarian/macrobiotic/etc.?**
  As far as I know, yes, especially if you already are. Some successful polyphas-ers have been vegetarians, vegans and raw-fooders. The only restriction seems to be that you really shouldn't be adapting to a new diet and a new sleep schedule at the same time—that's a common New-Years-Resolution-y thing that people seem to want to try, but it just never works that I've seen. Maybe people only have so much willpower, and each of those endeavors probably uses it all! ...I should also add, though, that there's no evidence that being vegetarian/vegan/etc. gives you an advantage in polyphasic sleep-ing, either. Some people claim that eating meat (or whatever) makes one's digestion sluggish or something, making polyphasic sleep difficult, but as the majority of successful polyphasers are still omnivores, I just don't think that can be true.

- **Can I drink pop/coffee/corn syrup/[insert unhealthy thing here]?**
  In moderation, it seems so. I drink coffee, but if it's more than a cup or two, it's decaf or half-caff. Too much sugar will mess me up, by making it difficult to fall asleep and then even more difficult to wake up; this was true before I was polyphasic as well, so I don't drink soda. You may want to seriously con-sider opting for low-caffeine and low- or no-sugar varieties of whatever your poison is, but you already knew you should do that anyway, right? Right.

- **What about huge meals, like at holidays?**
  Yeah, that's a tricky part for me—eating too much makes me groggy as heck, and sometimes it's very hard to wake up from the next nap. If you're well-adjusted, you may choose to sacrifice your efficiency today in favor of four slices of Aunt May's famous pie, and you'll probably recover just fine later on (as long as you stick to your schedule afterwards—don't let one goofed-up

nap cascade into many). If you're still adjusting, though, you may want to go lightly, since a big meal will really slow you down.

- **I regularly ingest some "other" substance that affects me physically; can I keep it up?**

  Okay, I'm using this space to simultaneously answer questions about prescriptions, herbal supplements, recreational substances, and what have you, because, lacking research on any of the specifics, the answers are the same: It's probably easier and better if you don't, but if you have to, be minimal and watch carefully for effects on your sleep; and if you're serious about adopting polyphasic sleep, be prepared to have to make some changes. (If you need a substance for medical reasons and can't make any change, be aware that this might be a deal-breaker. It's your call if you want to try anyway.) Some things are obviously more likely to be problematic than others – If you take tranquilizers or are fond of cocaine, you're going to have more trouble[70] than a weightlifter who takes creatine or a woman using black cohosh for menopause symptoms. A good rule of thumb is, "Does it affect your sleep now?" If so, the effects will probably be multiplied on polyphasic sleep, and that may preclude your being able to adjust or maintain the schedule. If it doesn't usually affect your sleep, it still might when you become polyphasic; however, the effects are more likely to be mild.

Note:

This is a new section in the Second Edition, because I've had much more experience, and many more discussions, about this topic since I wrote the First Edition.

Exercise & Athletic Lifestyle

When I started sleeping polyphasically in the year 2000, I got no real, regular exercise—I played on the school's ultimate frisbee team on and off, and went hiking in the mountains occasionally—but I was twenty years old and very busy, so I was pretty fit. When I re-adapted to Everyman, I was a more sedentary working parent; but around the same time, I began taking

---

70 Extreme examples, of course—at least in the case of the *abuse* of either of those substances, there'd be no way in South Cleveland that you could ever adapt. But you knew that.

Taiji classes. I became more and more attached to martial arts[71] in the following years, and as a result I began exercising more and more so that I could be in the best possible shape to pursue my art. In addition to a regular workout regimen involving weight-lifting, core-muscle conditioning and stretching, I've also become an avid swimmer. Having recently moved to an ocean-abutting city, I took up freediving, and then underwater hockey[72] and general swim-training so that I could be a better diver.

So initially my athleticism started very slowly, and I had only taken a handful of taiji classes by the time I was adapted to my Everyman schedule. I have re-adapted (after illnesses, travel, and my attempt to go back to monophasic sleep) in the years since, while my exercise quotient was at varying levels—but this may not be the same as adapting "from scratch" while maintaining an athletic lifestyle, so please take my advice with the appropriate quantity of salt.

Adaptation

I think it's pretty inarguable that the sleep-deprivation incurred during a polyphasic adjustment will almost certainly affect one's athletic performance negatively, and necessitates **extra care not to injure oneself** in any capacity. That includes:

- Injuries due to overtraining—pay attention to muscle soreness (which can be a symptom of polyphasic adjustment—see the section on Physical Effects) and be prepared to adjust or limit your workout. Don't be afraid to do less for a little while and work your way back up to where you were—that's better than how far you'll fall behind if you get hurt!

- Poor recovery (and thus a higher risk of injury later on) due to dehydration or protein starvation—if you train hard, make sure you get extra electrolytes and good burnable food at regular intervals.

---

71   Specifically, traditional Chinese Kungfu and Taiji—I blather about these pretty regularly on my website, if you'd like to read more about them.

72   Yes, a real sport; and freaking amazing—you should try it!

- Injuries due to poor form or concentration—on days when you are very sleep-deprived, I strongly suggest abstaining from workouts that require delicate balance and/or careful attention to form. No Crossfit, gymnastics or trapeze-artistry, for example. ☺

It's well-documented that during adjustment to a new sleep schedule, there's a period of mental and physical slow-down. It doesn't last long, but if you ignore it, it's the perfect place to injure yourself—think of someone who drains the oil out of their car so that they can replace it with newer, better oil. There's nothing wrong with the car having less, or no, oil in it for a short time, as long as the driver is con-scious of the fact that the car can't be taken on the freeway during that vulnerable period—it needs to recover first! (I'm pulling out the wild parable/metaphors and exclamation points because I know how gung-ho and competitive athletes can be. *Smart ones*, though, know when slowing down is in fact the best way to ensure that they're able to keep up the best performance overall—because nothing slows you down worse than getting injured!)

People who are already athletic, who plan to become polyphasic, should certainly **expect and prepare for a drop in performance**, and several weeks of needing to moderate and/or limit one's workouts. Exactly how much you need to slow down depends on your body, your lifestyle, and your sport(s) of choice—here, an athlete's increased ability to listen to their bodies and know their limits is crucial. Athletes who are either very new (and thus haven't built up the knowledge yet) or profes-sional (and thus have more to lose from smaller mistakes) should *definitely contact a medical professional* and arrange to have regular checkups as needed.

To the question, **Should Athletes be Polyphasic at All?**, I say this: It is true that sleep-deprivation impacts physical performance. Therefore it is true that the *adap-tation period* of adjusting to a polyphasic schedule will negatively impact athletic ability. However, since a polyphasic schedule does not involve *long-term* sleep depri-vation, it should not be contraindicated for athletes the same way, say, working 60 hours a week would be[73].

---

73 Yeah, see what I did there? I meant it, too.

After Adaptation

Outside of the issue of adaptation, polyphasic sleep still involves some special considerations for athletes.

- **Cool downs are important.**
  You won't sleep well if your heart is still thundering from a workout—make sure to leave time to get a shower or some other relaxing activity before you have to sleep.

- **Don't get too hungry.**
  There's a special kind of hunger you get from working out, especially when you started with an empty stomach; and it's almost impossible to sleep through. Make sure you have a small, easily-digested snack between a big workout and a nap.

- **Watch your recovery times.**
  If your routine banks on how long it takes your body to recover from torn muscle, be aware that polyphasic sleep may affect this. Some people have reported slightly longer recovery times (much longer, during adaptation), but others say theirs is unaffected, or depends on when they exercise relative to their naps. Everyman-sleepers may find that their body puts off muscle-recovery until the core nap.

- **Watch for unintended consequences.**
  Polyphasic sleep makes the kind of core change that can reverberate throughout your system in odd ways. As an athlete, you often rely on knowing precisely what your body's "settings" are, so make sure to watch carefully for several months, and don't ignore small things. If you're going to attempt any major feats, make sure you have a firm, recent assessment of where you are, in terms of energy, stamina, strength, balance, etc.

- **Be aware that huge workouts will necessitate extra sleep.**
  There is just no way that I can shore-dive for four-plus hours and then sleep four hours in the next twenty-four; *no way*. I've burned *over a thousand* calories doing that, and worked almost every muscle in my body to its limit, plus heaped on some serious mental aerobics too (in the form of survival

situations; the ocean is nothing like a pool in terms of mental and emotional activity). I can, however, have a 20-minute nap or two before bedtime, and then sleep for a somewhat longer core (4.5 or 6 hours), and be just fine. If I miss naps, though, I'm in for a solid 8-hour pass-out-on-my-face-a-thon. Since I don't do multi-hour shore-dives, or hockey tournaments, or similar activities very often, this isn't a problem; but it does seem to contraindicate polyphasic sleep for athletes who push themselves to the limit on a frequent basis.

Other than those tips, just remember that polyphasic sleep is a hyper-efficient method of sleeping, so treat it as you would a restricted diet. **For athletes, super-efficient diets are sometimes even more helpful than they are for others; other times, though, they're unworkable because they interfere with energy-levels too much**. Same deal here: Know thyself, and make changes consciously and with care. But if you're already awesome enough that you can be a hardcore athlete, I don't see what you have to fear from a little sleep-experimentation, personally. ☺

Deliberate Oversleeps/The "Crash Day" Theory

Every once in a while, someone asks me if polyphasic sleep should include a "crash day", usually interpreted to mean a day of (sometimes forced) long sleep – 8, 12 or even 24 hours' worth. As presented to me, this idea typically originates with a tale of one of the famous American scientists, who was reported to almost never sleep, but then would crash out for almost a full day once a week or month or something. As I've learned though, when it comes to pre-recording-device historical figures, sleep data is almost always speculation, and usually varies by source. The "scientist" in question here could be Edison, Einstein (who was German, though he lived in America for a time), or even Franklin, depending on who you ask.

It's also possible that this idea comes from an anecdote concerning one of Dr. Stampi's experiments, wherein after a month of successful polyphasic sleep (which, keep in mind, is barely adjusted), he tells his subject to sleep "as long as he wants" on a surprise day. The subject slept ten hours, after which he excelled on all his test-scores, and to the researchers' surprise, kept that performance-gain for some time.

This led to a theory that "sleep bonuses" could be beneficial in other circumstances. (The subject also returned to his Dymaxion-type schedule with no apparent difficulty.)

Source notwithstanding, I have no reason to believe that using a "crash day" is either wise or necessary *in normal circumstances*. For one thing, a well-adapted polyphaser, in normal circumstances, can't crash in the way that's described – to sleep that much would require having built up a significant sleep debt.

On the other hand, polyphasers who miss naps, or who burn a lot more energy than usual (see the section on "Exercise and Athletic Lifestyle"), may very well accumulate a sleep debt. Dr. Stampi's experiment, and some of my experiences as well, seem to indicate that taking a long-sleep day to replenish is a good thing, if one has built up a debt—though in the case of Stampi's experiment, I would argue the the debt he was sleeping off was very likely due to his still being in the adjustment phase (though granted, near the end of it... and the fact that he only slept ten hours agrees with that, I think; if he hadn't been adjusting, he would have had a lot more sleep debt than that, after a whole month of sleeping three hours a day!).

One interesting and related fact that seems to hold true: It seems that adjusted polyphasers with no sleep debt, when they "sleep in", can only sleep about 50% longer than their usual daily amount of sleep. When I was on Uberman, during the very rare occasion that I slept in, I would naturally sleep three hours (2h + 50%). I've heard this from other Ubersleepers as well. And now that I'm on Everyman, getting a total of four hours' sleep per day, if I decide to sleep until I can't any more, I typically sleep almost exactly six hours. Of course, if one were to keep sleeping in, especially in conjunction with skipping naps, that number would increase – but as far as one-day sleepfests go, the 150% ratio[74] seems to hold in general[75].

The concept of a *regular* "Crash Day" seems to be based on the reasoning that polyphasers are missing something which, if they let themselves sleep at will, their bod-

---

74    $n : n + (\frac{1}{2} * n)$

75   Does it also hold for monophasers? If so, it could explain why people who typically sleep 8 hours often oversleep to 12.

ies would "make up". Again, this isn't true based on everything I know. However, there are some possibilities for the truth of this that seem at least entertainable. For example, a "crash day" might be making up for missed:

- Laying down

- Exposure to darkness

- Closing eyes

- Slow, shallow breathing

- Slowing of mental activity

...I think those are plausible simply because yes, a normal monophasic adult gets quite a few hours of those things, every single day, and perhaps, though they don't seem necessary, the body needs them.

But if that's the case, would sleeping for half a day once in a while be the best way to make them up? I have found that I feel better, as a long-term polyphaser, if I wear a sleep mask during my naps (so that I get some darkness), if I prop my feet up and hang out on the couch for an hour or so a day (feels good to "lay" down for a while[76]), and if I meditate to drown out the constant brain-noise (but this was always true, whether I was polyphasic or not). But in the first year and a half of my Everyman schedule, I only slept for longer than six hours when I was ill; and I think I slept 12 hours once when I was really ill with a sinus infection in 2008. (In the intervening years since the Second Edition, I've had more breaks, including a deliberate attempt at going back to monophasic sleep, which there's a new section on. None of that has made me think that regular "crash days" are a good idea, with the exception of for athletes—see the section on Exercise & Athletic Lifestyles.)

In short, barring extraordinary circumstances that could build up a lot of sleep debt, **if you're on your schedule, stick with it**—that seems to be the best way to

---

76   See the section related to muscle soreness—"Long Term Physical Effects"

ensure that you get enough rest and sleep. Polyphasers whose schedules are regular and who are getting good rest don't need to, (and in my experience can't) crash for 12+ hours anyway. I suspect the "scientist figure(s)" who are reported to crash for long periods had simply been staying awake, or mostly staying awake, for days on end, as geniuses are known to do. ☺

If you *have* built up sleep debt and feel you need a "crash day" to make up for it, the following bears consideration:

- Sleep debt due to missed naps has already thrown off your schedule, and taking a long off-schedule sleep will throw it off further.

- Be extra careful that you get your naps on-time after a "crash day", and be aware that you may be unable to sleep for the first few, resulting in some sleep-deprivation feelings until your schedule evens out again.

- If you need a regular longer sleep due to strenuous activity or something else that has built up sleep debt (travel, illness, etc. are possible reasons for this—see the sections on those things for more details), then approach it consciously and with care. Remember that being polyphasic means being more productive/efficient at the cost of greater awareness of and control over your sleeping habits: A "crash day", if you decide to take one, shouldn't be an excuse for sloppiness.

Long Term Physical Effects

The question, "Are there physical effects to long-term polyphasic sleep, and what are they?" is a screechingly difficult one to answer right now. To know if there are side-effects that may present themselves to a significant portion of the population requires research, plain and simple. I can speak about it in generalities based on what I know from the reports of others, and I can speak to my own experience. Testimonials can be helpful to individuals sometimes, which is why I'm writing them down, but they're useless for developing a factual knowledge-base for the public. Hopefully there will be more and better information soon.

The physical effects of the adjustment period are fairly well-known (see the chapter on Adjustment). And barring research that can make more subtle determinations, it's fairly certain by this point that there are no, or at least no common, major nasty effects to living on a polyphasic schedule long-term. Buckminster Fuller did his Dymaxion schedule for two years while under medical supervision, and was famously declared "sound as a nut" by his doctor[77]. I've gotten regular checkups over the course of my experiment and I, too, seem to be fine. Neither I nor the others I've spoken with who've lived on Uberman for 6 months or more noticed any negative effects that seem to be a result of the sleep schedule itself.

So, to answer the naysayers, I think that based on what we know, and the research that's been done, it's safe to conclude that **long-term polyphasic sleep almost certainly does NOT cause**:

- permanent sleep-deprivation

- loss of mental acuity

- psychosis or personality change

- "debilitating arthritis"[78]

- physical deterioration (that we can detect)

...So that's as far as I'll go with "effects caused by the sleep schedule".

BUT changing a sleep schedule changes a lot else, and it's worth asking what those secondary effects might be, too.

Unsurprisingly, they seem to vary by person, but the ones I hear about a lot are almost certainly tied to lifestyle. Spending a lot of time on a computer, for example, has its own physical effects; and if as a result of your polyphasic schedule, you

---

77   See the Time Magazine article in the Resources section for the quote.

78   Yes, a commenter actually told me I would develop this.

spend even more time soaking in that lovely CRT (LCD, plasma, or whatever) glow, then you'll experience them more acutely and/or more often.

The major ones deserve individual treatment, I think. Here are some effects that I've had described to me by adapted polyphasers – that's not to say you'll experience them, or not experience others. But since they do seem to happen, here's some info on dealing with them:

Weight Gain and Loss

Reports of weight loss or gain aren't uncommon—I've actually experienced both. On Uberman, I was up and running a good chunk of the time I was awake, and often didn't eat until I was really, really hungry—I'd just get too busy, especially to stop by the cafeteria. By the end of the experiment, I was having to make a point of eating at least two large meals a day to stop the weight loss. (It wasn't dangerous, but you could see some ribs for a while.) Two large or five small meals would keep me at the right level. Conversely, when I adapted to Everyman, in the comfort of a well-stocked home, I gained a few pounds at first and had to put limits on my snacking. Eating does wake you up somewhat, but obviously it isn't wise to fall back on that too often!

Overall, people's eating habits generally change on a polyphasic schedule, but not much (unless you intend them too—but again, beware of trying to change too much at once). Being awake more often, you need to eat a bit more, or at least a bit more often, lest you do things like eat breakfast at 4 AM and then not get anything else until lunch at 1 PM. I prefer small, frequent meals anyway, so I just try to eat healthy and keep my portions small. The trickiest part is during adaptation: You don't want to deprive yourself, or make any major changes in diet, while you're adapting; and eating really is helpful for waking you up if you're sleepy. But you don't want to pig out and/or develop bad habits, either. I wouldn't see the harm in letting yourself snack as much as you want (especially if you stock up on healthy snacks) to keep your energy up, and keep you awake and comfortable, during the few really hard days of adaptation, though.

Which brings up an interesting point: There is an obvious possible secondary use of polyphasic sleep here, too, which hasn't really been explored. If you want to lose a little weight, you could adapt to a polyphasic schedule while making an effort to keep your eating habits, or at least your caloric intake, exactly the same. (I'm not sure if that would be particularly easy, mind.) Theoretically at least, you should burn more energy while consuming the same calories and thus lose weight (assuming your existing diet is balanced). I have no idea if anyone's ever tried this, and I wouldn't try it myself, since if you've got to count calories anyway, why not just eat less? Eating the same amount while being awake longer doesn't sound any easier than eating less, although I suppose there are circumstances that could make it so. Still, I would urge some caution trying this "polyphasic diet" hack with Uberman, since the weight loss seems to be at least potentially more dramatic, with more risk that it could be unhealthy.

One secondary use of polyphasic sleep that comes from this and is definitely positive is increased awareness of your nutrition: If you don't do it already, transitioning to polyphasic sleep can be a great excuse to start tracking your caloric, fat, carbohydrate, fiber, and protein intakes. For one thing, you'll have the extra time to devote to the tracking; and for another, if you see anything unhealthy going on, you'll be in a good place to make small changes to address it. (As many others have testified, oftentimes you don't even *need* to address it—the act of bringing awareness to what you're doing is often all the catalyst you need for change.)

Dry or Sore Eyes

Eye soreness is, as of the Second Edition here, a common enough complaint that I won't brush it off as "probably computer-related" and leave it at that, as I did in the First Edition. The truth is that most sore/dry eye-problems that people have during adaptation probably *are* related to spending more time staring at a computer-screen or television; when you have more time on your hands and need to fill it, that's often where it goes in this day and age. But even if you don't use a computer or watch a television any more on your polyphasic schedule than you normally did, you may experience dry or tired eyes, especially during the adaptation period. Here are several ways to prevent and treat dry and sore eyes:

1. Be aware of how much time you usually spend "staring at a screen" on your monophasic schedule. When you begin making the switch to polyphasic sleep, if your eyes become sore or dry, make note of how much

time you're spending staring at that screen now that you're sleeping less. If your screen-time has increased by even an hour a day, that's significant and could be causing the problem. Keep in mind that even the most dedicated nerds have to ration their screen-time somewhat. Everyone's personal limit differs, but if your eyes hurt, that's a good sign that you need to spend less time, or less consecutive time (see next point) in front of the ol' box.

2. No matter how much computer or TV-time you get, you should take breaks for your health. Every 15-30 minutes, make sure you stand up and walk away from the screen. Drink some water, take a bathroom break, do some stretching, or practice for a few minutes at another hobby. In addition to that, for your eyes' sake, always look away from the screen every few minutes, and focus on something distant. To help me remember this, I keep a nice picture or little sculpture within my line-of-sight while I'm working, and I've trained myself to stare at it when I'm thinking or stuck. (It was actually an eye-doctor who suggested that trick to me.)

3. Some dryness or soreness in your eyes is a common symptom of sleep-deprivation, so don't worry too much if you experience this during the adaptation period – it's normal and will probably go away in a few days, once the sleep-dep does. You can treat your dry eyes with plain saline eye-drops, or by putting a warm (not hot!) or cool wash-cloth over your eyes[79]. Standing in a steamy room or warm shower can help, too. When it comes to sore eyes, for some people, over-the-counter painkillers like ibuprofen help in the short-term; just don't overdo it or take them for more than a few days. If your eyes feel puffy or burn-y, try putting a cold pack (not too cold) over your eyes, or putting cool water in your hands and holding it over your eyes for a moment[80].

---

79   WARNING! Do not sit/lay down with a warm washcloth over your eyes if you're tired and shouldn't be sleeping! You'll go out like a light!

80   Also, slices of cucumber from the fridge look totally ridiculous, but they also feel *really good* on tired eyes. If it's late at night and no-one else is awake, who cares how you look, right?

4. If your eyes are sore / dry / tired, you may be tempted to sleep because everything else you do hurts your eyes. I've been there, too. Make sure you have a few things on-hand that you can do that don't require much from your eyes. Some types of physical exercise or practice can be done with your eyes closed, or at least not "engaged", as can some hobbies that you do with your hands (knitting, sculpting, playing an instrument, etc). Practicing things with your eyes closed, when you normally wouldn't, is also good for your brain (builds new neural pathways), and can be excellent for your practice of a particular art. But if you don't want to do anything that heavy, you can even just make a game of walking around your house with your eyes closed for a while, trying to memorize routes. (I've done sillier things to stay awake.) Think of a few things like this that you can do and write them down ahead of time, so that when your eyes hurt you can do something to give them a break without sleeping.

Sore Muscles/Body Aches

Like sore eyes, sore muscles and body aches are usually caused by the sleep deprivation during adaptation, or a "lifestyle" problem; and getting through adaptation or changing your behavior will usually make it go away.

When it's not just a symptom of sleep-dep, sore muscles sometimes mean that you're using the extra time gained by your polyphasic schedule to be on your feet and doing things more often. That was the case when I made my first transition to Uberman, and I was sore—the kind of sore you might expect from working out every day—for about a week, if I recall correctly. (This is also the adaptation I lost weight during, and the two may be—but aren't necessarily—related.) There's also the fact that you're probably spending less time laying down. For myself, this was a positive change; the soreness went away once I got used to moving around more, and I have much less neck and other "chiropractic" pain when I'm polyphasic than when I sleep all night. (I made "moving around more" a permanent goal as a result, and kept it as one even when I was monophasic again.) But depending on your situation, you may find that it disagrees with you to not have a long period of horizontality[81]. Sometimes, making a point of sitting back and putting your feet up more often can help—I did this when I was on Uberman, even after the soreness went away, simply because it felt good to recline and take the ol' gravity off. I do it sometimes on Everyman, too, especially at the end of a long—and by "long" I mean twenty-hour!—day. Depending on your age and physical constitution, you may find periods of physical rest more or less necessary.

Of course, sore muscles / body ache can sometimes be a sign that you're coming down with an illness, too. If you have a scratchy throat, a fever, or vomiting, you may be dealing with a case of the flu, in which case you definitely want to sleep as much as you can for a while (see the section on "Illness" under "Scheduling").

If your soreness is in your connective tissues rather than your muscles, this can be a sign of several things. It could be inflammation, which is caused by some chronic conditions (such as arthritis), some vitamin deficiencies, and for some people, any weakening of the system in general—meaning it could possibly be caused by sleep deprivation, too. Warm baths, gentle stretching, dietary or over-the-counter anti-inflammatories[82], and making sure you're eating well and getting lots of water (dehydration can really aggravate inflammation), can all help.

Based on what I know, the majority of problems with sore muscles or body aches will go away during the adjustment period, as your body adapts to the new routine. If you experience these symptoms and they don't go away within a few months, you may have to either treat them separately, or consider that perhaps a lifestyle with a hyper-efficient sleep-schedule isn't for you. Don't panic though—I haven't yet spoken to anyone who had to give up on polyphasic sleep for this reason.

---

81 It was either that or "horizontalness", which is ugly, or "horizontosity", which sounds like a brain-disease, okay?

82 Cherries have been shown to have anti-inflammatory effects in rats, and I know quite a few sportsmanlike people who recommend cherries or cherry juice for inflammation-related conditions. Just sayin'.

Cessation of Sleep Disorders

Will polyphasic sleep cure your sleep disorders? Well... to say that it does is a big claim to make, and I'm certainly not making it categorically, nor denying that it would need a lot more research to be actually substantiated. But I'll say that I have plenty of evidence that it *can*.

As with the rest of this book, I'm just telling what I know. The fact is that I know that polyphasic sleep (done properly) can have a positive, or even miraculous-seeming, effect on some sleep disorders. This may be because a large part of many sleep-disorders has to do with bad sleep habits, failed sleep rhythms, and general difficulties getting attuned to one's sleep cycle (or having one that isn't whacky). Adjusting to polyphasic sleep has, I think, the effect of erasing the entire white-board of your sleep-cycles and rewriting it from scratch, in a strict and therefore stable way. A stable schedule may not be a cure-all for sleep disorders, but it's not hard to believe that it helps, or that it might cure some people.

For me, the Uberman schedule "cured" the insomnia I'd been struggling with for months at the time. It also eliminated the nightly bad dreams, frequent night terrors, and bouts of sleepwalking / sleep-trashing-my-room I'd been experiencing (for most of my life, really). And when I say "cured", I mean that the very day I started actually being able to fall asleep for my naps and wake up from them without being a zombie – by day ten, maybe sooner – all of my sleep problems were gone[83]. As I said, I don't find this quite as surprising now as I did when it happened (shocked me to my toes then), but what I still do find surprising is that, except for the occasional minor instance, none of those sleep issues – some of which I'd had for many years – came back at all, not even during the periods when I went back to monophasic sleeping. That's partially why I think having my sleep schedule "wiped clean" and re-done from scratch may have been what did it. ...On the other hand, prior to trying Uberman, I had done plenty of things that I would have expected to

---

83 Actually, all my sleep problems were gone from the very first day, technically speaking. I didn't sleep for a few days, and was sleep-deprived for a week, but I wasn't having any (other) sleep-disorders either. Maybe what I should say is, "I've never had a sleeping disorder manifest during a 20-minute nap." Now that I'm on Everyman, I have had the very occasional problem with a nightmare during a core nap, but nothing I would call a "disorder".

reset my sleep-schedule too, including making small and large adjustments to the times and durations of my sleep, and purposefully staying awake for days at a time. Those, though, had little or no effect on my sleep problems.

Regarding actual sleep disorders at least, I've spoken to other people whose frequent nightmares, morning exhaustion, sleep movement and other problems disappeared when they adapted to a polyphasic schedule. (I've never spoken to someone who had apnea and tried polyphasic sleep, so I can't speak to that.) And it would certainly seem that polyphasic sleep, if other factors don't contraindicate it, is a pretty safe thing to try, if you have one or more sleep disorders. Personally, I'm in favor of trying any kind of lifestyle change that might work to cure a problem, before resorting to drugs. The only caution I'll offer[84] is that, while properly adapting appears to sometimes have these wonderful effects, "experimenting" without the necessary strictness (failing to adapt) can make many sleep problems even worse, by throwing off what schedule and good habits you did have. So if you have one or more sleep disorders and are interested in trying polyphasic sleep to alleviate them, be responsible and be sure you plan your adaptation carefully.

And lastly, added for the Second Edition is this paragraph, because someone told me that they expected the section on "Sleep Disorders" to cover sleep disorders that polyphasic sleep might *cause*. The only thing I have to say on that, though, is that I've never heard of one. I suppose you could count the people who try and fail numerous times to adapt, and in doing so, ruin their sleep-schedules and sometimes need drastic measures to get back on a schedule... but they have a disorder that wasn't caused by polyphasic sleep per se, but rather by trying to do polyphasic sleep the wrong way. I'm not aware of any polyphasers developing sleep disorders they didn't have before.

Dreaming

This section belongs right between the ones on Physical Changes and Psychological Changes, I thought. ☺

---

84   ...again...

Much of what happens regarding dreams is individual, but there are a few things you can probably count on: For one, **you will probably stop dreaming during the beginning of the adaptation process**. This is probably a physical effect of sleep-deprivation, perhaps due to the fact that when you are managing to get to sleep, you're falling straight into a very deep sleep. The not-dreaming will last until your body begins to get accustomed to the naps. Most polyphasers consider "dreaming again" to be a good sign that their adaptation is progressing.

Also, almost everyone I've ever talked to notices an **increase in the vividness** of their dreams, when they first begin having them again. I was no exception. I'm unable to determine whether this vividness is caused by the strictness of the schedule, the exactness of the amount of sleep had, recovery from sleep deprivation, or other factors; but I am fairly certain that it isn't caused *only* by sleep deprivation. The reason for that conclusion is that, now that I'm adapted, if I miss naps or end up very tired, I sleep very heavily and generally don't remember my dreams. I call this "zonking"—if I get very tired, I have a nap where I just seem to shut off like a light-bulb and wake up a bit disoriented, rested but feeling like it's only been seconds since I went to sleep. Dreams return to being clearer and more memorable when my schedule is on-track. (It might be accurate to say that sleep-deprivation is the cause of vivid dreams *during the adaptation phase*, however—further research would be required to make any real claims about it.) The vividness in dream-recall tends to decrease once one has been polyphasic a while, but by how much is up for debate. (I'm not sure how you'd quantify it anyway!) I typically have several dreams that I can remember every day, and while it seems to me that I can remember them clearly, it's hard to say how clearly you remembered your dreams several years ago (can you answer that question?), so as to whether they're still as vivid as they were, I'm afraid I don't know.

Dreams can seem omnipresent, too, for the first few months of being polyphasic. Part of the transition into a polyphasic lifestyle is getting used to sleeping many times a day, and that means getting used to *dreaming* many times a day. This can be weird at first, since your dreams often don't seem any shorter when they come during naps (in fact, many of mine felt longer)[85]. It may also be easier to remember your dreams, because you wake up so soon after going to sleep. I've gotten used to having (remembering) between 2-4 dreams a day, and this doesn't mess with my head anymore—but during both of my adaptations, I remember thinking it was really weird at first. Like having a second life! This is made even more striking by the occasional "ridiculously long dream" that polyphasic adapters often report having—a dream that seems to last for weeks, months, or even years of subjective time. For my part, I tended to have these before I was ever polyphasic, and I had quite a few of them during the adaptation process, but they've lessened in frequency since. In general, it seems that dreaming, like many other functions, gets shaken up during the adaptation process, and settles down (though not exactly the way it was) once you're used to the new schedule.

Also, some people on Everyman report that their body seems to "learn" to do its dreaming during one specific nap, often but not always the core nap. As with most highly-individual things, if the way your dreams are happening isn't bothering you or ruining your life, it's probably fine!

Lucid Dreaming

Lucid dreaming is a fascinating phenomenon that involves achieving a degree of wakefulness without interrupting a dream. There are a great many people who have an interest in this phenomenon, and most of them wish to bring it about more often. (Anyone who's had one will probably understand why—they can be insanely cool.) Because lucid dreams tend to happen more readily when the body is stressed or the sleep is unusually deep and/or fitful (which are also circumstances under which we tend to have very vivid dreams), it's been said that sleep deprivation may help bring about lucid dreams. Sleep dep, as well as other methods for unbalancing the body, are sometimes used as temporary measures so that a practitioner can have a few lucid dreams and then, if they know what they're doing, learn to recognize them and bring them about in normal sleep.

---

85   This might also contribute to the time-dilation effect [see next section] – when you're having what feels like 4-6 days' worth of dreams every day, it's easier to lose track!

Many people report an increase in lucid dreaming activity during the beginning of their adaptation, during or just after the adjustment period. For people who aren't familiar with the phenomenon, it can be a very powerful and/or unsettling thing to suddenly have lucid dreams—they are, however, totally harmless as far as I know. The occurrence of the occasional lucid dream during the adjustment period is not surprising; and moreover perhaps we should be glad there's some perk to act as a silver lining to the ickiness of sleep-deprivation!

Several people I've conversed with have told me, with great excitement, how useful polyphasic sleep could be, if you were really into lucid dreaming and wanted to work on it. For one thing, you'd have up to six chances a day! Also, maybe a poly-phaser's vivid dreams, which sometimes persist even after adaptation, are a sign that lucid dreaming would indeed be easier to bring about on a polyphasic sched-ule. Unfortunately, I've never known anyone who's primarily used polyphasic sleep for that. From what I know about lucid dreaming, it's probably difficult enough that trying to master it while simultaneously becoming polyphasic is just too much.

My recommendation, which you should take with a grain of salt since I'm no expert in lucid dreaming, is this: If you're interested in studying or experimenting with lucid dreaming, I imagine it would be more useful to get the hang of the basics of lucid dreaming first, and then do your polyphasic adaptation (preferably to Uber-man, Dymaxion or Tesla, for maximum effect) afterwards. "The basics" include get-ting used to writing down your dreams immediately upon waking, and developing a routine of asking yourself a trigger question, such as "Am I awake?" on a regular basis. (Google will give you much better information on how to learn lucid dream-ing, if you're interested.) And for goodness sake, if you pull off using polyphasic sleep to "crack" the trick of summoning lucid dreams regularly or even more than a few times, please let me, or one of the other Polyphasic group-maintainers, know!

Psychological & Social Effects

There's no way I'm going to be able to cover all of the possible effects here, so forgive me in advance. Being polyphasic does many, mostly subtle, but definitely interesting things to your mind. For the most part, they seem to be neutral, with a few positive and a few negative possibilities lurking in the wings. If you take good care of yourself, all the evidence I know suggests that you should be just fine (or better off) mentally as a result of adopting a polyphasic schedule.

Sleep is a different animal when you get it in small chunks. Some of the ways in which this manifests are obvious immediately; others take a while to notice. And I think it's difficult to appreciate how huge a chunk of your life sleep is until you make a big change to it. (People who take up fasting will say the same thing about food; and people who walk across the country will say it about walking. Challenging your perception of how something you took for granted really impacts you is part of the self-discovery process.)

Naturally, the effects of making such a change will differ from person to person, mind to mind. With that in mind, though (har har), here are some guidelines and general truisms:

Changes in the Perception of Time

Some things are predictable and seem to happen to nearly everyone: A shift in how time is perceived is one of them. Sleep plays a big part in how we mentally divide up our days! It can be hard to remember, or understand, that time is entirely a product of the human mind; but boy will drastically changing your sleep schedule remind you of it.

Time Dilation is the most common, and I think the most striking, effect: Days get longer, far more than it seems like 4-6 extra hours can account for. Sometimes they seem to last for a week! When I was on Uberman, I frequently asked what day it was, got an answer, and replied, "What, still?", or was genuinely worried for a minute that it was *next* Monday already and my homework was late!

Naps, too, dilate greatly—one 20-minute nap can seem like it lasts hours—though most people get used to that part, and after a while, naps no longer seem as ridiculously long as they used to, except for the occasional one. Someone posited to me that naps can seem so long because your brain is used to a certain amount of time passing while you're asleep (especially when you wake up fully rested), and this certainly sounds like a plausible explanation. Either way, it can be disorienting when it happens, but most people seem to think it's nifty overall, to wake up feeling like they've been asleep for many hours, and to find out that only 20 minutes have passed.

The other thing that can happen to one's perception of time is that it can seem to simply go haywire for a while. It's not unusual to need "backup" help keeping track of time for the first six months, primarily and especially on Uberman-type (equi-phasic) schedules. Watches and calendars are your friend!

Also, when doing Uberman (or, as I hear from others, Dymaxion), it can be amaz-ingly hard, even well after adaptation, to figure out if it's night or morning, and of what day: Is it dark at 5 PM or still dark at 5 AM? Is this midnight going-into-Monday or coming-out-of-Monday? When exactly does it stop being Tuesday and start being Wednesday, if you're basically awake for all of it? It's hard to explain what this feels like to someone who's never done it, but try to imagine: after several weeks of no "long sleep", your experience becomes that of living *one great big long day*, with no discernable end to it. On the one hand, it's super cool—sort of like a feeling of immortality, or unstoppability—but on the other hand, it can get confusing, even if you're wide awake and thinking perfectly clearly. I was deftly handling homework and class and work and scheduling of all sorts, and not falling behind at all, but still having trouble keeping track of the days without constantly asking people!

I solved that problem eventually, by the way, by giving names to the nights—I picked an arbitrary time for the day to end in the evening and a time that the new day should begin in the morning, and then named the periods between the days. (I had a list called "Times of Darkness", and it was such wonderful, pseudo-poetic col-lege stuff... I wish I still had it!) This made it much easier to keep track, as opposed to just trying to notice a single switch at midnight.

On Everyman-type schedules, dilation is still sometimes an issue, but losing track of days is usually not much of a problem—you have that long core-nap to split your days on, and for me that's always been enough. The individual days still feel awfully long sometimes—and sometimes I experience a sort of "psychological tiredness" (maybe it's emotional in nature?) because I feel like I've been going and going for so very long; I will find myself thinking, "Holy crap, is it *still* Monday?" in the wow-it's-been-Monday-a-long-time sense; but I don't get *confused* about what day it is. I wake up from my core at 4am, and it's a new day; easy. Hopeful equiphasers should be prepared to adjust for the loss of a day-marking sleep-time, though.

Euphoria

This is doubtless one of the weirder effects. I'd have discounted it as "experimentation glee" or a bit of a manic phase on my part, if it weren't for the many people in the years since who've reported the same effect. This only seems to happen with Uberman[86], but it seems that polyphasic sleep can cause a sustained state of mild euphoria. It doesn't make you "high", to be clear. (Well, at first the sleep dep will, but that's not a high most people find enjoyable. I certainly didn't.)

This euphoria is a sense of very sharp clarity, of fluid mental acuity, and in general feeling at ease—literally, as if things are easy. It is, to be cultural and silly a moment, somewhat like realizing you're in The Matrix: Everything slows down; you feel like you're functioning much faster and better than the world around you. For me, this feeling came and went for several months, sometimes sticking around for days at a time. I've heard roughly the same reports, not from everyone, but from the majority of people who adapted successfully to Uberman, and notably, from *all* of them who adapted successfully the first time they tried to. (I have no idea what a first-try adaptation has to do with it, but literally everyone I've known who's pulled one off[87] has reported the euphoria. Non-first-try adapters seem to experience it less often. Maybe the build-up of sleep debt, or habituating the brain/body to equiphasic living, plays a part?)

The euphoria is great, as most euphorias are. However, if you're just in it for the consciousness-polished-to-a-mirror-shine feeling, you might want to reconsider: Uberman adaptation is *really* hard to pull off, and while I (and others) think it's worth it for what it can do overall, it probably isn't worth all that trouble just to feel zingy for a while. (Learn to meditate instead; it's a much more direct route!) But that zingy feeling sure is a nice reward for all the hard work.

---

86   Some reports of a similar effect have come in regarding Dymaxion and Tesla, but it's hard to compare since so many more people have done Uberman than those two.

87   Not that that's very many people.

Changes in your Social Life

Your social life is almost certainly going to change when you adopt a polyphasic schedule. I've already mentioned that if you're a Party Hard or Type A Workaholic type person, you may have problems adjusting to the need to "put the world on hold" every couple hours and sleep—and this is probably true of anyone who leads a very world-immersed life. On the other hand, if you take a break from your fre-neticisms[88] while you adapt, and then go back to it with your new schedule in place and your new needs in mind, even a hectic lifestyle might not be a problem.

Something to watch out for, though, is that whether you do or don't lead a particularly hectic life, you're probably going to end up spending a **greater percentage of your time alone** than you might be used to. (If your life is super-busy, you may be able to just fill in all the time you gain from your new sleep-schedule doing what you normally do. This is not typical, however: Most people end up with at least some free time that they have to spend alone.) If you don't have a solitary hobby or three to make this time pass more easily, you may want to go get some.

If you go out often with friends, you may face another interesting problem: **Social-circle friends** aren't always the kind of people you want to have deep discussions about your lifestyle with, so you may feel uncomfortable telling them about why you have to go sleep in the car for twenty minutes at midnight. Proto-boyfriends-and-girlfriends, which loose social groups tend to contain a lot of, can be very judgmental and sensitive to things which look socially "weird". This could be a real problem, for some people. If I were asked for advice about that type of situation, though, I would say, the opinions of half-strangers aren't worth changing how one lives one's life over; and all the people that you actually want to spend time with are going to be cool with you doing the kinds of things with your life that you want to do—if they're not supportive, or can't take how "weird" you are, then there are better fish in the sea. Confident people who let go of relationships that don't support who they want to be... end up with better relationships. So if being polyphasic is something you want to do, but you're worried how your social circle will take it, I suppose the question you face is, "What's more important to me—doing what I want, or making sure people like these see me as acceptable and nonthreatening?"

---

88   Ssssh... that's totally a word.

Also, if you have **family** around, you may have to adjust to spending a bit less time with them overall—you're going to take an hour or so worth of naps during the day, and make up for it with several hours of available time that'll usually come while everyone else is asleep. Some people have found that this makes them lonely, or doesn't work with their family life. You'll definitely want to talk to your loved ones about it before you do it, and discuss how you'd like to address that change. You may have to make a little conscious effort—to play with the kids, or spend meaningful time with your spouse—to make sure you still get an acceptable amount of valuable time with your family. However, that's sort of true of Life anyway; there's almost always something trying to get in the way, and it's our priorities and our efforts that make the difference. Being polyphasic hasn't negatively affected the time I spend with my family, but that's because we've all worked together to make sure it didn't. ...And just like regular sleepers, sometimes I go tired so that I can do something with my kid. I think every grownup does that. ☺

Learning to Love Sleep

Many people who adapt polyphasic schedules do it at first because they have some degree of difficulty getting a good, monophasic night's sleep. Some, like myself ten years ago, have gotten to the point of simply hating sleep, and wanting as little to do with it as possible – and if you've had sleep-troubles for a long time, this is, I think, a perfectly normal way to feel.

However, on a polyphasic schedule, once the icky adjustment part is over, you may find yourself liking sleep again. The reason is that you'll have gone from trying to sleep at one time per day and (to some degree) failing, then feeling tired for all or most of the rest of the day; to feeling tired at specific times, and answering that feeling with immediate, restful sleep. Even the most die-hard sleep-haters usually find themselves with a different opinion, a few months in: **Suddenly it feels good to sleep**; it directly addresses and cures your tiredness, and it's painless (maybe much more so than you were used to), and it doesn't even take long!

The warning here is to beware sleeping in because suddenly you like to sleep— disliking sleep can make adaptation easier, because you don't have much urge to oversleep; but then, when you stop disliking sleep, you can sometimes find yourself fully adapted but having to fight off the psychological (pleasure-driven) desire to sleep. Talk about cruel ironies!

Being A Weirdo

Being seen as a weirdo is nothing new to me, so I tend to gloss over that effect; which is why I'm making a point of mentioning it explicitly here. If you sleep poly-phasically long enough, you *will* get some attention over your schedule, whether you want it or not. You can hide it, but since being polyphasic involves napping during the day, it's likely to come up eventually, and you're going to get peppered with questions and probably judged a minor lunatic at least a few times. Now, I'm hardly a social juggernaut, but I've learned to smile and shrug it off, so you probably can, too[89]. But if you don't want to have to, then definitely think twice about being polyphasic. If you just want to have all such conversations over with as quickly as possible, consider memorizing or carrying a short description of polyphasic sleep (like the one in the Cheat Sheets section) that you can deliver on-demand. Some people may still want to ask questions, but lots of them won't.

Just in case they help anyone, here are some of the things I've learned to say, to brush off or minimize the "Look, it's a circus freak[90]" effect. Mind you, in a perfect world we would all smile and say, "This works for me—what of it?" and never apologize for anything... but the real world isn't perfect, not all of us are comfort-able confronting the curiosity of the masses head-on, and there's no harm in the occasional white lie or misdirection if it saves you some trouble and doesn't hurt anybody, right? Right.

If confronted, try saying:

---

89   This may be too flippant of me: I not only have a lot of practice being weird and shrug-ging off the social difficulties of it, but in recent years—especially the post-First-Edition years—I've made a *huge* effort to become more adept socially; and to that end, being polyphasic has been both a challenge and a big help, since it presents me with a lot of sink-or-swim opportunities.

90   Not that that's a bad thing; circuses (circii?) can be awesome, and many freaks've got mad skills!

- *Nothing better than a good nap!* (if you don't have to admit to *only* napping—this way you don't look any weirder than anyone who's ever taken a nap somewhere, and that's most people.)

- *Bah, sleep is for the weak!* (if you do have to admit it—I find that throwing in a "I'm off my rocker and thrilled about it" grin will get most people to mumble something inoffensive and scurry away asap. Call this the Ford Prefect defense. ☺ You can also try quoting Ben Franklin, "There will be sleeping enough in the grave!", or make up a witty retort of your own. Just remember, if it's *too* witty, you may get stuck explaining it.

- *It's just an experiment I'm trying* (add "for school", "for a friend", "for my doctor", etc. as you feel you need to, for legitimacy—people are less weird about an "experiment" that has some external cause... which is a pretty funny attitude especially in countries supposedly devoted to individualism and personal freedom, isn't it?)

- Or, if you get caught napping somewhere you don't often go, you can say *I'm just not feeling well.* This has always worked for me in a pinch, when I need to get people to leave me alone about it, stat. This is actually my stock "oh-look-I'm-in-some-random-parking-lot-sleeping-in-my-car-and-somebody's-decided-to-knock-on-my-window" response. It'll even get policemen off your back!

...Or (and this is probably healthiest in the long run) you can just get used to being a weirdo. It's good for you—helps you appreciate your own individuality. If it's practical, I highly suggest just going ahead and being weird. (For one thing, I need the company!)

Readjusting to Monophasic Sleep

This is a new section for the Second Edition, since I've made several attempts—mostly short, but one of three months—to return to monophasic sleeping in recent years.

So as not to keep anyone in suspense: I *hated* it.

When I'm monophasic, I feel the lost time keenly. On Everyman3, I have 2-3 hours of time to myself in the morning (starting at 4 AM) to work on my own projects before work; and I can stay awake fairly late. Even on Everyman 4.5, when I have to be in bed by 11:30 to wake up at four, I feel like I have adequate time for my work and practice. But when I'm monophasic, I either have to be in bed at an outrageous 8 PM in order to wake up at four—meaning I have no evening at all—or I can stay awake until 10 or 11 PM, and sleep right until I have to get ready for work! I find doing either of those things on a regular basis soul-crushing, not to put too fine a point on it.

I also *loathe* waking up after eight hours asleep—I'm stiff, and groggy, and my brain doesn't want to boot up without coffee. If there was tension in my shoulders or neck before I went to sleep, I'll wake up sore, too.

Difficulties re-adjusting

In my experience, re-adjusting to monophasic sleep is pretty painless, and can be done over a few days. When polyphasic, I don't sleep eight hours by default, but if I start leaving my alarms off and sleeping as long as I want, plus skip my naps during the day, I'll quickly start sleeping longer and longer at night.

I do experience some sleep-deprivation, especially during the day if I'm forcing myself to not take a nap; but since monophasic is about more quantity rather than efficient high-quality sleep, the sleep dep wears off after 3-5 days of crashing all night.

Every time I've been monophasic after my very first experiencing as a polyphaser in the year 2000, I've felt that the quality of my rest was reduced, the quality of my waking-time reduced, and overall the quality of my life not as good as it was when I was polyphasic. (I've also always felt that the quality of my life was *highest* when I was on the Uberman schedule, and that it's slightly less good on Everyman, but still quite a lot better than when I'm monophasic.)

Default schedules ("Permanent Adaptation")

I've been asked if Everyman has become my default schedule, or if I think polyphasic sleep could become someone's default—or, to put it another one, if one could "permanently adapt" to polyphasic sleep.

I'll start the answer by saying that I believe that the human being is inherently a programmable thing, and I've witnessed plenty of stranger defaults than polyphasic sleep. Like most habits, sleep-habits seem to be more deeply ingrained when they're:

- taken on earlier,

- persisted in longer,

- supported by lifestyle, and

- are a good fit with the constitution and design of the hardware and software ("person", in the parlance) that they're running on.

So yes, I'm quite sure it's *possible* to become a default-polyphasic sleeper: probably to some degree in almost everyone, given enough effort; and to greater or lesser degrees depending on the individual and the circumstances.

I would not say that *my* default sleep-schedule is (yet) polyphasic, though of course defaults are not binary values, and I'm definitely not "just" a default-monophasic sleeper constantly holding my monophasism at bay anymore, either. If my lifestyle is stable and I'm putting in the minimal amount of effort needed to get my naps, I find polyphasic sleep easy[91]. Yet, probably due to some combination of my decades of early training as a monophasic sleeper and my lifestyle's tendency to be very informed by the monophasic schedules of the rest of the world, I will, if I stop paying attention to my sleep-schedule, begin sleeping longer at night and taking less naps.

---

[91] I should say, I find *Everyman* easy, because it fits my lifestyle right now. I'm pretty sure sustaining Uberman would be more effort—but that isn't going to stop me from doing it the second I think I could manage it!

I start to feel poorly about the time I hit one nap a day and six hours' sleep; and then I have to either get another daily nap and cut my core to 4.5 hours (I find Everyman 4.5 pretty comfortable, though I don't like it as much as Everyman 3), or get more sleep at night, in which case I'll either stop napping or my nap will become less restful, and wham, I'll be monophasic again.

However, I don't find it comfortable anymore. Interestingly, even when I was monophasic for months at a time, I continued to get a little bleary at the approach of my naptimes, and to crave naps at the times I was used to taking them. Sometimes I *would* take them, and I'd feel better for it. This may be because I wasn't sleeping as well monophasically, too; it's hard to say. I definitely felt less rested more of the time on a monophasic schedule than I do on a polyphasic one, so even if monophase is my default, this is an instance where I'm willing to put in the effort to work against my default state in order to live and feel better.

Behavior also makes a big difference in what your easiest schedule is, and I have some learned skills that make me more comfortable / normal a polyphaser now. As long as I'm not under undue stress, I can very quickly will myself to sleep, especially at naptime[92]. I can set a pretty reliable "mental alarm" for "about 20 minutes" and wake up reliably between 15 and 30 minutes, depending on circumstances. (If I'm sleeping in a comfortable place and my schedule has been regular for at least a few days, I can almost bet on hitting nineteen minutes every time.) Oddly enough, I can also set a mental alarm for "about 20 minutes" when I'm not sleeping, and it usually works pretty well (and comes in surprisingly handy sometimes).

Of course, being polyphasic gives you some skills that are *not* terribly handy to have as a monophaser, either. For instance, I'm super comfortable sleeping in my clothes. Given the option, I tend to prefer sleeping bags over blankets (though actually I think I did that as a kid too, so it may just be a prediliction, and not directly related to how much time I've spent snoozing in a sleeping bag in a car). I don't always associate "morning" with "shower and brush teeth etc" and if I'm not having

---

92   This is a skill that most polyphasers who've been adapted for at least six months
       tend to develop.

a really regular schedule life-wise, I'll need to set alarms to make sure I do those things at the appropriate intervals.

One last word on defaults: I believe that it's beneficial for everyone to learn to control their defaults, and to choose, wherever possible, which behaviors are their immediate unconcious preference. This is a hugely powerful way to exert control over your circumstances, and where it's easy—like with the little things—there's just no downside that I can see to making it conscious. Now, some defaults are easier to modify than others, and for many people "to control" some things may go farther than "accepting that this is how it has to work for me"—and that may include sleep, which is definitely not a small or inconsequential habit. And if that's the case, I say that's fine; being eyes-open about something that's not worth the huge amount of effort it would take to change is absolutely a form of conscious control too.

But we are by and large changeable creatures—programmable, as I've said—and I think it's healthy when we recognize this. I also think an attitude of "I chose this" is a very positive thing to have, and so **I always try to encourage myself and others to choose what's in their power to choose, and choose to accept what isn't**: This leads to minimal flailing and whining, which waste energy and make people unnecessarily miserable.

Habits and defaults are some of the most powerful things that affect our daily lives. Your habit of (say) eating some junk food in the evening can *radically* change how you look, feel, and act, especially over time—think of how different a person you'd be after ten years of that, versus ten years of a different habit, like taking a short run every evening. The effects of even small habits are HUGE.

Sleep is not a small habit: it's one of the very fundamental ones, and as such, it's not easy to change. But the effects are *massive*. Polyphasic sleep is definitely not a beginner's course in habit-changing and default-control, but it is, I think, one of the cooler options for those who aspire to Epic Self-Hackery.

VIII.   Philosophical Implications

What are the philosophical implications of polyphasic sleep? This is probably a little-addressed question because for many people, the phrase "philosophical implications" causes instant heartburn—and that's fine, but I'm not one of those people; I love philosophy. So, while it's perfectly alright if others don't care to read or ponder this section, I am, in the grand tradition of philosophers everywhere, going to write it anyway. ☺

The first question to be addressed is, of what kind are the philosophical implications that a sleep schedule might have? Traditionally, sleep has had something of a "monkeywrench effect" on many theories of consciousness; it makes a great example to bring up whenever someone claims something akin to Descartes' "I think, therefore I am"—oh yeah? Do you stop existing when you sleep?—or posits any theory that doesn't take our periods of personal darkness into consideration. Philosophers have argued about whether sleep constitutes being totally blacked-out and gone, personhood-wise; or whether the mind might retire to some other realm by itself; and what these different views of sleep mean for their pet theories of consciousness[93]. In these cases, though, sleep is a philosophical tool rather than its subject, and I think there's room for it to be a subject, too. Specifically, I think that sleep, especially with the advent of polyphasic sleep as a possible long-term schedule, raises ethical questions, specifically when it comes to the normative value of[94] sleep.

---

93   If you're interested in reading more about how different philosophers have batted this issue around, there's a paper I can recommend, which I enjoyed and thought gave a good overview of at least the classic Western philosophers. It's *The Philosophy of Sleep: The Views of Descartes, Locke and Leibnitz*, by James Hill, published in the Richmond Journal of Philosophy in Spring 2004. I will admit right now that I'm not as well-read as I'd like in theories of consciousness specifically, so I apologize if I've missed something obvious.

94   A fancy way of saying "goodness or badness of"

Is it morally good to sleep as much as one wants? Should we restrict our sleep if possible, striving for regularity and efficiency rather than indulgence; or does sleep, as an involuntary bodily function, merit indulgence whenever needed (like having to pee)? There's a popular view, more assumed than stated, that sleep should be indulged in whenever possible, for as long as the sleeper wants (within reason, which people seem to define as something close to the normal average range, or more for sick people); and that it should, ideally, not be subsumed to efficiency or other concerns. But there's also a separate assumption, informed by asceticism perhaps[95], that to freely indulge in even "normal" physical demands is damaging, or at least likely to hinder higher development of the mind and spirit. Despite our tendency to trust some assumptions inherently, there isn't solid evidence either way, and you can see expressions of both of these opinions—both the sleep-indulgence and sleep-restriction proponents—everywhere.

We know that being sleep-deprived for long periods of time is unhealthy (a fact that's often utilized by the sleep-indulgence camp), but that doesn't help us judge the ways of restricting sleep that don't cause long-term sleep deprivation—like polyphasic sleep. People who "train" themselves to sleep less, or who are able to sleep very little naturally, or who sleep on odd schedules to maximize their efficiency, are viewed with a mixture of admiration and concern. What are we concerned about? Simply their health, or is there something more fundamentally "wrong" with not sleeping the usual amount, that we don't know how to express yet?

On the flipside, we also know that moderately restricting food intake—caloric restriction—is healthy, and in fact might even extend one's lifespan. Perhaps overindulgence in sleep is no more healthy than overindulgence in food. But again, what is overindulgence? If you could sleep 6 hours per day on a schedule that included napping, and be healthy, is sleeping all night for 8 hours too much?

---

95   Remember that not only Buddhism, but Christianity too, was partially based on ascetic (deprivation-based) traditions.

It all comes down to how you view the purpose of sleep, I think. Here are some views that I've espoused or considered in the course of pondering the subject:

One possible view: Sleep is a mechanical recharge, like plugging a batteried object into the wall for a few hours. There's something about sleep that either connects us to an energy source, or allows the mind/body to generate extra energy and store it for waking use.

The normative implications of this view favor restriction, *if* restriction can be done in a healthy way. If you're recharging your batteries, doesn't it make sense to do it in the most efficient way possible? Would you refuse an upgrade to your electric car that made the batteries able to charge faster? Living—being awake and aware—is pretty much an unqualified good, so to have more of it must be good, and if all that's in the way of that is mechanical efficiency, then restricted schedules which work are not only "a good", but it becomes almost a moral imperative to adopt them if possible.

There are a few problems with this view, though: One, as we learn more, our bodies are seeming less and less like simple machines. To assume that we're built to run (be awake) during only 2/3 of our available time due to a simple need to recharge our batteries every day seems overly simplistic, maybe even increasingly unlikely, the more we learn. (Then again, maybe sleeping all night is a genetic or evolutionary throwback, like our pinky toes; or maybe it's just a habit we learned for some ancient social or survival reason and are now stuck with a physical dependence on.) A second problem is that this view invites negative judgment of those who sleep any more than they must, and that smacks of a sort of Puritanical nastiness. Overindulgence isn't good—I agree with that, in general—but when it becomes morally necessary to restrict oneself beyond the natural tendencies, all kinds of mean and judgmental behavior towards others, far more negative in its effects than an individual's overindulgence, can result.

A second possible view: Sleep is an experience with its own inherent value, perhaps of a spiritual or consciousness-related, rather than physical, nature. Maybe sleep is time we use to connect with the Void or the Great One; perhaps we lose waking consciousness while we commune with the Eternal and Infinite[96]. Maybe our minds get in the way of this communion[97], and need to be "shut off" so another part of us can do its thing. It's been suggested that we're built to put our minds under for a while each day so that our [souls / subconsciousnesses / essences / pick a word] can connect with the [Source / Void / God / collective unconscious / pick a word]. And while there's no firm evidence (duh) to support such an idea, there isn't any to really disprove it either, since modern science currently doesn't "go there".

But assume that it's true—that sleep is there for a reason all its own, for some nonphysical purpose that can't be made more efficient through sleeping in naps. On this view, it's no longer morally desirable to restrict our sleep just because we can—indeed, it becomes akin to skipping church, or maybe something even more serious, like skipping drinking water—to do so. To thwart such a connection may be to do damage to what we fundamentally are, cutting off a part of our lives that's as vital and necessary as the waking part. Indeed, to weaken or restrict such a connection could even be doing damage to us on a level we're not yet equipped to understand: Perhaps, just for a fun conjecture, sleep is how we stay "in contact" with the place/state we came from, and not getting enough can hurt our chances of making it "back" after we die[98].

Of course, this view relies on a whole bunch of assumptions that, even if I wanted to take the time to try and prove them, I probably couldn't do. If you happen to believe them, then maybe you can choose to believe this about sleep... but even then, you won't have a clear answer as to what to do about sleep, either. Perhaps the sleep you get on a restricted schedule is enough. Perhaps no sleep is enough unless "done properly", and how to do it properly is anybody's guess. Maybe sleep has an even deeper purpose still, which we simply haven't figured out yet! ...This is a pretty enough view, but it has a rabbit-hole in the middle, I think.

---

96   Or call it what you want: the important thing is that some other *type* of consciousness is going on, which is itself important for our functioning or development.

97   To wit, Adam could not survive hearing the voice of God?

98   Dibs on the sci-fi plot!

Then there's also a third option, which is to take the first view and give it a twist: Maybe sleep isn't really necessary at all! Maybe it's an evolutionary artifact that we can overcome, or will eventually "grow out of". This view is supported by stories like that of Thai Ngoc[99], the man who mysteriously lost the ability to sleep, and has lived for 33 years without it, and apparently boasts a clean bill of mental and physical health.

If sleep wasn't necessary at all, would you still do it? How many people do you think would continue to, for how long? Do you think it would eventually be consigned to the category "Wastes of Time"? ...Or, to ask it another way, beyond the fact that we (seem to) need it, does sleep have any real value?

Would you give up sleep? If I could never sleep again and never be tired, I would probably try it, but I can also see myself regretting such a decision, finding in the future that I couldn't tolerate "being here", in the world, 24/7. Maybe sleep exists to keep us sane by giving us a "time out" from what is otherwise a complicated and often emotionally brutal existence. Food has a "comfort" element that would prevent us from wanting to give it up entirely, and for most people, sleep does too... the major difference is, I think, that restricting one's food intake, within reason, is generally accepted to be sensible and healthy. (Food is also a finite resource that we must share, however. We can't all sleep all the time, but within reason our over-sleeping doesn't hurt other people.)

This is a major problem, though: With most things, if there's no clear-cut answer one way or the other, it's best to side with Aristotle and aim for "moderation in all things". But **what's "moderation" when it comes to sleep**? Sleeping until you're only a little tired? That's courting long-term sleep deprivation, which is the one thing most people (scientists and polyphasers and moms alike) agree is the least desirable of the outcomes! With sleep, it seems that the only sensible options are to either sleep until you're completely refreshed, or to restrict sleep to the least you can get and not be tired (which seems, for our purposes, to entail a nap-based schedule); and neither of them are obviously moderate.

---

99   Among other places, you can read his story here:
      http://www.thanhniennews.com/features/?catid=10&newsid=12673

This little twist makes sleep one of the hardest items of personal care to build an ethical view of. We know we should bathe and be as clean as possible (within moderation); we know we should eat what we need to live and so that we're not hungry (within moderation); we know we should exercise and keep our bodies in good repair[100]. But how should we sleep? A whole lot, so we're not tired, or very little, so we're efficient at spending our time (since now we know that this can be done without being tired as well)?

Fortunately for me, it's beyond the scope of this section to pick an answer; and anyway, from where we stand, to do so would be arbitrary and premature. **There are philosophical implications to polyphasic sleep, insofar as it's opened up the possibilities**. Instead of "sleep a lot" or "be sleep-deprived," our choices now include "put in some effort to sleep very little and not be sleep deprived". And that means we're all stuck pondering whether this is morally a better choice for those who can make it, and how much, if at all, those who don't sleep polyphasically ought to be trying to.

Thankfully, I enjoy pondering. If you do as well, your thoughts on this topic would be a welcome addition, so write them down (If I can do it, you can do it.)

---

100   Yes, again, within moderation—Lots of exercise is good, but exercise taken to extremes is not healthy either.

IX. Conclusion

...And that's all of it, really. Some appendices (stuff I didn't know where else to put, basically), resources, and contact information follows; and you can always find more on my website, as well as a lot of embarrassing blow-by-blow of my mistakes and realizations in the archives. Also, if you purchased this book, keep your receipt, since there may be later "editions" (there's no plan for a Third yet, but you never know) and if you show your receipt, I'll give you an electronic (PDF) copy of any of the editions later than the one you bought for free. (I don't believe in forced obsolescence, hmph.)

Speaking of (even) further editions, if you know of any information that isn't contained in this book which should be, please contact me through my website at http://www.puredoxyk.com and let me know about it? While the amount of information on *polyphasic* sleep is (at this moment) scarce, it's developing quickly. (Sleep itself is another matter. You can tell that I've tried to restrict this book to being about polyphasic sleep, rather than sleep in general, simply because I didn't want it to be 43,000 pages long.) You can also use the website to tell me about your personal website or blog that has to do with polyphasic sleep. (Such things are a bit too ephemeral for a book, I think.)

As for my **final comments on polyphasic sleep**, well, obviously it's been a positive thing for me, overall. I won't say it hasn't been difficult, nor will I say that the extra waking-time I have doesn't come at a price: Getting here was hard; and I definitely have to "watch my sleep schedule" like some people have to watch their diets, and I probably will for as long as I live polyphasically.

Polyphasic sleep is a lifestyle change, and it's had a surprising range of effects on how I live.

- I've become more organized, more aware of my priorities, more attentive to my body, and more appreciative of what my time is worth.

- These experiences have also taught me a lot about sleep, some of which I'll always be glad to have learned:

  - I know how to tune my mind and relax my body so I can fall asleep in minutes, and I can wake up refreshed less than half an hour later. (Some people claim that after a time, you just "learn to nap", like riding a bicycle. This has been my experience. It's also been my experience that my "napping skills" can be sharper or duller depending on what my schedule has been like recently, and other factors.)

  - I can, barring extraordinary circumstances, set a "mental alarm" and wake up without assistance in about twenty minutes.

  - I know what environments I can and can't sleep in.

  - The difference between good, refreshing sleep and bad sleep is like day and night[101] to me now—before polyphase, I thought I knew the difference, but I didn't.

  - I know how to recognize when I'm tired, and how tired I am, and when being tired is affecting me physically or mentally. Again, I thought I knew these things before, but it turns out that I didn't, not really.

The mind and body are amazingly complex and subtle things, and I'm glad to know more about how they work together than I would have, had I not undertaken these experiments.

---

101 I'd like to apologize for that, and all the other, puns and linguistic goofiness in this book... I'm just a sucker for such things, plain and simple. ☺

I wouldn't have written this whole thing if I didn't see a benefit to others in polyphasic sleep schedules. Not to everyone, of course; but to a significant minority at least. I used to think that maybe this idea would change the world – maybe it would be the beginning of a 24-hour society, of more flexibility for working people with families, or of a global appreciation of how important getting good sleep and using our time well is. That all may never happen, of course. Maybe all we get out of polyphasic sleep in the long run is that some people gain a new respect for time and our mind/bodies, and a boatload of extra time to pursue their hobbies in for a while.

I think that would be fine by me.

Thanks very much for reading!

~"PureDoxyk" (Marie)

http://www.puredoxyk.com/
puredoxyk@puredoxyk.com

X. Appendices

Appendix I: Sleep Drugs

One can hardly write anything this size on sleep without mentioning drugs. Personally, my take on pharmaceuticals has always been "Not unless I bloody have to"—I read a lot of science fiction, and I'm fundamentally uncomfortable with a huge industry that draws insane profits off of people's illness and, when that's not enough, turns to producing drugs for people who aren't ill and profits madly off *that*.

That's not to say "drugs'r bad, m'kay" or that I haven't or wouldn't like others to benefit from medical science, but I do think our society turns to drugs way too often and without proper consideration for the long-term consequences; motivated, as we are, by an endless marketing blitz that often reminds me of something out of a Philip K. Dick novel. When people give kids psychotropics to control their behavior without ever considering whether that six cans of Coke a day is having any effect, I want to punch them. ...All of which is entirely my opinion, of course, but it never hurts to know the bias of your author.

With that in mind, I've never taken a sleeping pill in my life[102]. I try everything else before I resort to drugs for any condition, as a general rule; and it was in the midst of "trying everything else" to fix my sleep problems in college that I stumbled upon polyphasic sleep, which, for me, did the trick. (And it's a good thing, too, because it's unlikely that sleep drugs would have been a good idea, or an efficacious one, for dealing with what I was facing back then.) I think that makes me uniquely unqualified to discuss the various substances that are prescribed to cure or sleep disorders, or improve the quality of sleep or wakefulness for people who don't sleep well for one reason or another. I do know that this class of drugs can often be addictive and/ or dangerous if taken improperly, in excess, or in combination with other substanc-

---

102   Except for melatonin, which I tried a few times with no effect.

es, so if it's a route you or someone you know is pursuing, then please, hit the books hard and be vigilant.

However, there is one sleep drug that I have read up on pretty well, and which is interesting for being in a different class from the rest of the stimulant/depressant drugs, and that's **modafinil**. Modafinil is marketed by the drug company Cephalon in the U.S. and UK as Provigil[103], and in other places as, generally speaking, Moda-something or Something-vigil. It's been around since 1998, and it doesn't appear that there will be generics until at least 2012. Modafinil's intended use is as a treatment for narcolepsy, though it's prescribed off-label for ADHD, depression, "shift-worker syndrome", sleep apnea, vague complaints of daytime sleepiness, to help with the fatigue-related symptoms of MS, Parkinson's, chemotherapy... and quite a bit else. The "point" of Modafinil, as I gather, is to make sleeping about 6 hours as restful as sleeping about 8 hours, and to keep the fatigue caused by sleep-deprivation (or an illness) at bay. (Update: There's a derivative / new version of this drug called Armodafinil, marketed as NuVigil, too.)

I have no personal experience with Modafinil, but I have talked to some people who have, and among other things, I've read an excellent piece that Slate.com published[104], wherein an author takes the drug for a test-drive and reports some interesting and lucidly-considered results. He seems to experience minimal physical side-effects, but a powerful and immediate psychological addiction. And I wouldn't be at all surprised to know that addiction results from a drug that allows its taker to feel like they're "cheating sleep"[105]. Obviously, if Modafinil (and probably similar drugs as well) can be addictive—and we don't know if it can be *physically*

---

103 I agree with the people who've called this name "Orwellian" and "creepy".

104 Which you can read here: http://www.slate.com/id/2079113/

105 Some have even described the Uberman schedule as "addictive", for the same reason I suppose.

addictive—then the long-term effects should be better known before such drugs are made widely available. The last thing we need is millions of people hooked on something that later turns out to be deadly (*coughcigarettescough*).

I'll say one more thing on the topic: Sleep is part of a balance. You expend energy; you must recover it somehow, and the standard way (but maybe not the only way?) is by sleeping. The polyphasic schedules in this book do not let you "cheat" sleep—they let you trade some of the duration of sleep for frequency of sleep, at a cost of some effort and planning. The result is that, overall, you sleep less, and you pay for it by sticking to your naps (which isn't such a bad price, according to some of us). *Drugs don't let you cheat either*—**there really is no way to cheat; a balance is a balance**. Even if you could "meditate instead of sleeping", which seems to be a popular way-out-there alternative, you'd pay for it by spending years, possibly decades, learning how. In the case of drugs, they let you trade some sleep-time, sleepiness, or difficulty sleeping, for certain effects on your body—long and short-term. This trade might be worth it in some cases... but it would be pretty ill-advised to make that deal without knowing exactly what you're trading for, unless you're in a desperate situation. I can see using sleep drugs occasionally as being possibly worth it; with something like Modafinil, and medical supervision, you can be fairly certain that the short-term effects won't be too bad. I would even be happy, as a consumer, to have the option to have something like Modafinil in my house in case I felt I needed it (and you could argue that I do: it's called caffeine... however, from all the available evidence, Modafinil works better against sleep-deprivation symptoms than caffeine does, and of course caffeine can be strongly physically addictive too).

But I wouldn't use it, or any other sleep drug that I know of, with any regularity or for a long period of time, unless I had some condition that made it worth the possibly-serious, unknown long-term effects. Using drugs to alter fundamental physiological responses should *always* be done with caution, and with the assumption that those responses are there for a reason. (Yes, I mean to say that sleep-deprivation symptoms are there for a reason. But remember, polyphasic sleep isn't trying to cheat sleep-dep; it's enduring a bit of it to switch schedules, and after the switch it goes away on its own.)

Appendix II: Arguments to Bosses

Convincing a boss to accommodate your polyphasic schedule can be tricky—how tricky depends largely on your job and who you report to, secondarily on how much has to change in order for you to be accommodated, and thirdly on how well you present your case. Here are some tips for pulling off the last one:

- Know exactly what you need, and be prepared to state it in simple, clear terms. "I'd like an extra half hour for lunch, which I'd be happy to make up by coming in half an hour early. I would spend the extra time in my car, sleeping. I have a timer so I know I'll wake up on time," or, "I'd like permission to close my door from two to two-thirty, turn off my phone, and take a nap."

- Make it sound serious, unless your boss is the type to appreciate quirkiness in hir employees (hint: most aren't, so if yours is, you probably know it). A good approach may be to explain that you have a terrible time sleeping normally, it's affecting your work, and you'd like to try a possible solution you learned about.

  - Don't explain all about polyphasic sleep, unless your boss seems interested. It just sounds weird to some people. Instead, simply say that part of the solution involves taking a nap at X time.

  - If you can say with any degree of honesty that you've discussed it with your doctor, do; any degree of medical-establishment involvement makes a powerful argument to workplaces.

- Offer to do something to compensate for any off-the-clock time your schedule will cause. But if you work for a smaller business and are paid hourly, also offer to *not* make up the time, since saving half an hour a day's worth of your pay may sound good to your boss.

- Be prepared to answer questions about where you'll keep your blankets, how you'll keep people from waking you up, etc. Bosses are often anxious to know that your napping won't be disruptive, and showing that you've thought it all out helps.

- However, don't spout off a bunch of details without being asked, either. State your case, make your request, and then *wait* for a reply. (This is an old ~~Jedi mind~~ sales trick—It's harder for someone to say "no" when they're engaged in the conversation, as opposed to listening to a lecture.) Answer the questions you're asked, and ask some of your own if you can, to keep the conversation two-sided.

- If you can, have your blanket/timer/pillow/etc. handy, so that if your boss asks about them you can show them to him/her and explain where you'll be keeping them. (I wouldn't suggest walking into the boss' office carrying them though!). The thought of a blanket in a place of work can give bosses the heebies—seeing a small, neatly folded one and hearing that it'll be in your bottom drawer or in your car can allay that response.

  - Do not, however, show off "scary"-looking things like your timer, your sleep app on your phone, or the ducky you snuggle with. ☺

- If you have trouble, consider seeking out a sympathetic doctor. This works best if you actually have a sleep disorder, but some doctors will write you a note saying they approve of your attempting a nap-schedule if you tell them you're having trouble sleeping and would rather try polyphasic sleep before you resort to drugs. (Which may even be true, like it was in my case.)

  - You can, as an alternative, just ask your/a doctor to write you a note saying you need a nap during the day because you're frequently exhausted and you think it'll help you normalize your sleep-schedule... skipping over the issue of polyphasic sleep altogether.

  - Also, sometimes just telling your boss that you're trying to avoid taking drugs to help you sleep is helpful. Nobody likes drugged-up employees; they tend to miss work.

- If you're really serious and your immediate boss won't hear of it, consider gently bringing it to the attention of the next-higher-up. Avoid saying anything at all negative about your direct supervisor unless you feel it's worth making your work-day miserable over; but sometimes telling a bigger boss that you think your request is reasonable, and that it would mean a lot to your feeling positive about your job, can help. Bigger bosses often work in words and numbers more than in people, and an easy way to keep your "performance" and "job satisfaction" high might appeal to them.

    - Don't go crazy and ask everybody up the chain of command, though, unless you want to risk being seen as a nuisance.

- If it seems your boss won't budge, don't push—shelve the issue for a little while, and bring it up again later, at a time that's favorable to you (during a review in which you did well, for instance). If you're a good worker and gently insistent about wanting time for your nap(s), they might decide to indulge you because it's a cheap way for them to keep you happy.

Appendix III: Sleeping in Public

Sleeping in public can be looked-down upon, in some places and by some people, and usually for reasons that I consider pretty dumb. On the upside, though, if you're only sleeping for 20 minutes, the chances that anyone will actually wake you up during that time to force their opinions on you are pretty slim!

If you are interrupted, try to be polite of course, but in my opinion one shouldn't be apologetic: What you're doing may seem strange to some people, but that doesn't make it wrong, and unless you were actually causing a disturbance or getting in someone's way (in which case, do apologize, even if it was unintentional), then it was at least as rude of *them* to wake you as it was of you to be sleeping wherever you were.

Whether and how you sleep in public is going to be mostly determined by **where you are**, I think: In Boston, people taking naps on the grass in parks or on benches next to the water is totally common, and I'd do it without a second thought—I've never seen anyone have their person or things messed with as a result of catching a cat-nap. Then again, this is a wonderfully polite place, and when I lived in the Detroit area I wouldn't have *ever* considered sleeping out in the open without someone to watch over me and my stuff.

Colleges, I've found, are also really friendly places to nap; though obviously being a student or having some other legitimate reason to be there makes it better, especially indoors. Not only did I sleep all over the place at St. John's, but I've seen many sleepers at or near the University of Michigan campus in Ann Arbor; people dozing in Harvard Yard are not uncommon at all; and on a recent trip I crashed on a padded bench in a hallway at Carnegie Mellon (where I totally was not a student or anything) and didn't get so much as a sniff from anyone (thanks, CMU!). So if you're not sure where to sleep and you can find a campus, I highly recommend it.

Libraries and bookstores, if big enough and possessed of couches or comfy corners, or even better, staffed by someone you know, are good options; **bars, restaurants** and **coffee-shops** that don't mind are too. Some people consider this rude, but personally I don't see anything more disruptive about pausing to snooze for 20 minutes on a bench or against a wall than anything anyone else is doing there, as long as it's either okay with the owners/employees or not causing them any trouble. (Should everybody do it all the time? No, but if we got to the point where many people needed to, I'm sure some enterprising folk would invent locations just for napping. Until then, nappers are a tiny population and unlikely to cause problems with their numbers.) Do be aware of ways you might be being rude, though—don't nap in a store or library if you snore, for example; and if it's a for-profit establishment, especially one being nice to you by letting you snooze somewhere, make a point to buy something at least once in a while.

More guerilla-esque are the **big box stores**, and I'll say right up front that I have zero love for these monstrosities and what they do to communities for the express purpose of siphoning money into major corporations' pockets; and thus very little sympathy for whatever arguments their purveyors can make that they shouldn't be slept in by people, especially if those people also happen to be part of the local population and thus paying for that store in terms of poor land and energy usage, decreased job-quality, crappy health insurance and benefits coverage for their neighbors, terrible product-quality and customer-service, immoral outsourcing and generally horrendous business-practices. I haven't had to do it myself, but I see nothing wrong with using one of these increasingly-ubiquitous places as a short-stay hotel if that's your best option: I'd look for low shelves where you can get behind the merchandise, or a display area for beds or furniture (though I wouldn't sleep on any of the furniture; too obvious—get under or behind it instead). Of course an employee will wake you and make you leave the store (oh darn) if they find you, but especially during off-hours and overnight, it's plenty easy to be ignored for thirty minutes. Go for it.

If you can sleep in a moving vehicle (and just because you can't while monophasic doesn't mean you won't be able to while polyphasic), **a public transit** trip is sometimes a good, cheap option, especially in the wintertime when parks, lawns and benches are inhospitable. Avoid rush hour, though, and if you're carrying a bag or gear, get it tied to you or tucked under you, just to be safe.

When I had a **car**, I often found it my best possible place to nap outside my home: It was warm(ish), private, and with a little work, comfortable enough (which of course depends on the car. The least comfortable thing I've ever tried to sleep in was a Volkswagen Bug!). Again, though, it does depend on where you are: In Detroit I could pull discreetly to the back of a (free, empty) parking lot (again, for only about 30 minutes total) for my daily nap, and at least once a month a cop would bang on my window, or some creepy passer-by would (often a creepy male passer-by, and/or one looking for a handout—but also sometimes one who thought I needed help for some reason, or who thought that their status gave them the mandate to police who was parking in the empty sections of their lot and why). After a while I began hanging a sign on my window that said, "Just napping for 30 min", and that stopped the passers-by, for the most part, but not the cops. Go figure.

Airports are great if you happen to be in one, but usually so remote that getting to one isn't helpful. If you're small/skinny you can often nap on the chairs, though I'm a big fan of just laying on my luggage on the floor; I can almost always make that comfortable. And of course, nobody messes with sleepers in an airport; it's awesome.

Generally speaking, **in more rural areas I would be more careful**, unless of course you're rural enough that you can be assured of being completely alone the whole time, in which case go nuts. ☺ It's definitely true that there's safety in numbers, especially for short periods of time; and places with lots of people engender good behaviors like "ignoring things that aren't your problem" and "generally not messing with people unless you have to". In my experience, overall, small towns and suburbs are worse places to nap than cities; and open farm-country, while peacefully empty, does carry a higher risk that if someone finds you, they'll give you some variety of shit.

On the subject of **signs**: Some polyphasers I know have favored holding or setting up a little sign explaining that they're just grabbing a catnap. (I'm always reminded of Granny Weatherwax's "I AINTN'T DEAD" sign. ☺) Whether you prefer to do this depends, I think, on how much you want people leaning over/near you to read the sign, and how frequently you think you'll be woken/interrupted without it. I used them for my car as mentioned above, and I love signs for my office door—I put up a sticky note that says "Please do not disturb ~ 20 minutes" and that works perfectly—but I don't think I'd use them if I were just sleeping in the open somewhere, since it's a common enough sight here and I think I'd attract more attention with the sign than without it. I can see having a sign that said "Polyphaser" being a useful thing once it's a more well-known habit, though!

Lastly, **gear**: Napping in public is greatly aided by having the right gear. If your polyphasic schedule assumes at all that you'll be sleeping "abroad", be cognizant of what you can carry compactly to make things more comfortable. Most people's phones can now function as white noise generators and alarms, so that's easy (set it up before you need it though; fiddling with your phone when you're tired and propped against a wall and time is ticking is not much fun); an eyemask is small (and easy to improvise out of a sleeve-of-something; I've done that a lot); many people can sleep without a pillow, or improvise one out of anything-that-fits-under-the-back-of-your-neck. Be cognizant of whether you need ear-plugs or any other special gear to be comfortable enough to sleep well! My biggest challenge has always been the blanket: Even in summer, I'm just not comfortable without something covering at least part of my body, and a blanket is a tricky thing to carry. In cool weather, I've had great luck with a long coat—my wool trench-with-a-hood is fantastic as a blanket—and when I've had a car, I always kept a sleeping-bag in it. When I've have no car, if I was out and planning on needing to sleep, I'd bring my bigger backpack and carry my packs-incredibly-tiny-for-travel sleeping-bag—setting it up and repacking it would be several minutes of work each, but it'd be worth it for the increased chance that I'd sleep well (and no harder than schlepping a regular blanket). In time, I may buy a travel blanket just for this purpose, though.

Appendix IV: Refutations

Have there been any refutations—formal arguments against—polyphasic sleep? Actually, yes, there have. The most comprehensive one I know about was written in 2005 by a Dr. Piotr Wozniak; you can read the entire (huge) paper online, here: http://www.supermemo.com/articles/polyphasic.htm. Dr. Wozniak covers most of the common arguments against polyphasic sleep in his paper, as well as some, er, "unique" ones.

You can read my refutation of Dr. Wozniak's paper on my website, here: http://www.puredoxyk.com/index.php/2006/11/01/an-attack-on-polyphasic-sleep/. I pointed out the bad facts (there are several) and some of the unsupported assumptions (ditto), and took issue most strongly with the fact that Dr. Wozniak considers all the blogs about *failed* polyphasic attempts as crushing ironclad evidence that no polyphasic attempt can work, but then stridently, openly ignores any of the same type of evidence that claims that polyphasic sleep *can* work.

Dr. Wozniak is pretty well-read in sleep issues, and he is an advocate for another alternative sleep pattern, which he calls "free-running sleep". (It's basically exactly what it sounds like.) And while I don't doubt that sleeping whenever you're tired would be nice, I've also dubbed FRS the only less practical sleep schedule than Uberman that I've ever heard of. I simply can't imagine a situation in which someone with any responsibilities whatsoever could pull that off.

However, I should mention that Dr. Wozniak himself is a very respected weirdo, and a lot of what he's written, I found to be both creative and well-informed; and where not, at least really interesting. I certainly wouldn't attempt to discredit him or his body of work as a whole. It's just unfortunate that he seems to have had an agenda, and a lot of bad information, when it came to writing about polyphasic sleep. I'll call it a very good day indeed when/if we can change his mind.

Appendix V: Resources

Here's a collection of some of the resources that I found useful for researching, adapting to, and continuing my education about polyphasic sleep[106].

Articles & Blogs

The **Google "polyphasic" Group** at http://groups.google.com/group/Polyphasic is a great place to start; their archives are a phenomenal resource. The group is loosely moderated (I help, along with several others) to avoid spam, but do be aware that, as is often the case on the Internet, sometimes people in this group who really don't know squat go spouting off their opinions; if you read something extraordinary, be sure to double-check before deciding to believe it.

The Polyphasic Wiki is an excellent general information source: http://polyphasicsleep.info

There's a new, but already pretty thriving, **polyphasic community** website, with articles, fora, and all-hours chat, at http://www.polyphasicsociety.com/. I'm really excited that things like this are beginning to exist!

Steve Pavlina's Polyphasic Sleep articles are one of the best blow-by-blow descriptions of an Uberman adaptation out there, although I don't believe his experience of being able to move naps as far as he does is typical: http://www.stevepavlina.com/blog/2005/10/polyphasic-sleep/

The **Wikipedia Article** on Polyphasic Sleep has some good information, and is missing other good information (par for the course with Wikipedia, yeah? ☺): http://en.wikipedia.org/wiki/Polyphasic_sleep

My First Writeup – the **Uberman's Sleep Schedule Node @ Everything2.com**: http://www.everything2.com/index.pl?node_id=892542

---

106 Note: This is not a bibliography for this book; I used in-line citations rather than a bibliography here. This is simply a collection of generally useful resources.

Sleeping Schedules is a collection of articles on different schedules: http://www.sleepingschedules.com/

BBC Article about using Polyphasic Sleep in Solo Sailing: http://news.bbc.co.uk/1/hi/uk/1180274.stm

Dr. Claudio Stampi

New for the Second Edition is this collection of links to Dr. Stampi's work, which is more well-represented online now, and worth its own research for those who are very interested in the science behind polyphasic sleep. The more I learn about Dr. Stampi, the bigger a fan I am—the angle he's approaching polyphasic sleep from is different from mine, and very practical in its own right; and the quality of his work is *very* high. Thank you, Dr. Stampi!

The **Chronobiology Research Institute** in Cambridge, MA was founded by Dr. Stampi as the *Sleep and Alertness Research Center* in 1990. It doesn't appear to have a webpage, but questions can be directed to info@chronobiologyinstitute.org.

Video Documenting Stampi's Uberman experiment:
http://www.youtube.com/watch?v=myi2sRph69A
Note, this segment is from an episode (show 105) of the excellent old PBS program "Scientific American Frontiers" (with Alan Alda! wow, memories). This episode originally premiered on Feb. 27, 1991. You can read a transcript of it at: http://www.pbs.org/saf/transcripts/transcript105.htm#5

This **Sample Data from one of Dr. Stampi's studies** is very informative concerning both the type of information gathered in chronobiological research (still a very new field!) and the type of studies Dr. Stampi conducts: http://www.sitesalive.com/ocl/private/04s/sleep/slp040608.html

Wikipedia Article on Claudio Stampi:
http://en.wikipedia.org/wiki/Claudio_Stampi

Wikipedia Article on the book Why We Nap:

http://en.wikipedia.org/wiki/Why_We_Nap:_Evolution,_Chronobiology,_and_Functions_of_Polyphasic_and_Ultrashort_Sleep

Further Research

The Stanford Online **Archives on Buckminster Fuller**:

http://collections.stanford.edu/bucky/

Original **Time Magazine Article on Buckminster Fuller:**

http://www.time.com/time/magazine/article/0,9171,774680,00.html

Journal of Clinical Investigation study on Sleep and Growth Hormone (warning: hurts to read, but very informational in general):

http://www.pubmedcentral.nih.gov/articlerender.fcgi?artid=436797

The Supermemo (Dr. Wozniak) **Article Attempting to Disprove Polyphasic Sleep:**

http://www.supermemo.com/articles/polyphasic.htm

(My rebuttal:

http://www.puredoxyk.com/index.php/2006/11/01/an-attack-on-polyphasic-sleep/)

Transcript of Video Spot on "Nap Salons" and **why naps benefit working adults**:

http://www.healthology.com/sleep-disorders/sleep-disorders-news/video4247.htm

Detailed article on **ProVigil** (modafinil):

http://www.healthology.com/sleep-disorders/sleep-disorders-news/article1258.htm

Slate.com **Reporter's Personal Experiment with ProVigil** (modafinil):

http://www.slate.com/id/2079113/

Extensive (very enthusiastic) **New Scientist article on Modafinil:**

http://www.newscientist.com/article/mg18925391.300

Tools

Typing Master online typing test/speed clocker:
http://www.typingmaster.com.au/java/ttapplet.htm

Online "Simon" Game (for testing memory & reflexes):
http://www.thepcmanwebsite.com/media/simon/

Alzheimer Association's Comprehensive Tests (speed of thinking):
http://cognitivelabs.com/alz_assoc_refertestpage2.htm

Placebo's Blog – home of the Sleep Track mp3s and software to track naps:
http://www.placebo.serv.co.za/

Polyphasic Society Chat Channel:
An all-hours IRC channel for polyphasers—in my experience, a friendly crew and a great place to go for questions, help, and general just-keep-me-awake-ness!
http://forum.polyphasicsociety.com/chat/

About The Author

Updated for the Second Edition (because the Author is just as new and improved as the book):

"Puredoxyk" is a batty woman named Marie who recently moved to the Boston area. She looks vaguely like this:

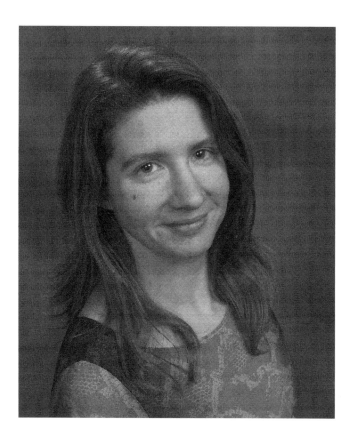

...and lives by five self-written commandments, which you get to read because they're the author's answer to "If you had very little space to say anything, what would you say?":

- Keep Trying

- Pay Attention

- Have One Intransitive Faith

- Doubt Everything Else

- Love Anyway

...Having said that, though, it also bears mentioning that the author is a passionate lover of words (scifi! philosophizing! songs!), martial arts (Kungfu! Taiji!), swimming (freediving and underwater hockey!), logic games, computers, pliers, airplanes, and oh yes, *learning as many new things as will fit and doing them as hard as possible.*

You know that story about the old lady who picks up the violin for the first time in her eighties and winds up first chair in an orchestra? That's about me, shortly after I invented time travel. (Because come on. Sleep-patterns that break the perception of time are only the beginning! ☺)

XI. "Cheat Sheets":
Things to use for reference

Following are some Quick Reference pages and parts of pages, for you to cut or tear out, copy and paste, print and fold up or hang up, and generally in whatever way is helpful use, to kick-start your brain on some key aspects of the polyphasic transition. Just so you know, I didn't use anything of this sort when I adapted—all I had was a friend, a timer and my Big Fat List of things to do with the extra time. But there were many requests for "Cheat Sheet"-like objects, and if they help some people out, wonderful.

As with the rest of this book, if you have suggestions for improvement, send 'em along via my website. I've also tried to leave lots of room on these to write your own notes, additions, etc. Happy Napping!

Why I Want to be Polyphasic:

Here or on another sheet, write down all the reasons why you want to be polyphasic. State your case loud and clear, and then keep this with you to remind yourself why you aren't going to give up!

☑ **Reasons to be Polyphasic:**

_____

_____

_____

_____

_____

_____

_____

_____

_____

_____

_____

_____

_____

_____

_____

_____

_____

_____

_____

_____

What is Polyphasic Sleep?

Here's a "cheat sheet" for those of you who want an easy way to describe to others what you're doing. Someone suggested memorizing a version of this; someone else advocated making copies to hand out to curious bystanders—it's up to you, of course.

❶ What is Polyphasic Sleep?

Polyphasic Sleep is an alternative sleep schedule that aims to be more efficient than "monophasic", or "all-at-once-at-night" sleep. In a polyphasic sleep schedule, several naps are taken throughout the day instead of one big "nap" at night. Done properly, this can reduce the overall sleep needed per 24 hours from eight hours to four, or even two, hours total. Many people have successfully used polyphasic sleep this way, sometimes for long periods of time, including the famous scientist Dr. Buckminster Fuller, and it appears to have no ill effects. Getting used to a polyphasic schedule means being pretty sleep-deprived for a week or two, which most people find difficult; but the sleep-deprivation goes away after adjustment. Polyphasic sleep also requires a very strict schedule for the most part—naps have to happen on time, and if a polyphaser misses a nap, it can be as tiring as missing most or all of a night's sleep.

Get more information at: ubersleepbook.com

When You First Wake Up

The time immediately after waking is a crucial one, because if you're tired, it can be very easy to talk yourself into going back to sleep "for just a few minutes". Adapted polyphasers would do well to avoid this habit, as it reduces the efficiency of the schedule and can lead to tiredness (or even ruin an established schedule); and for new polyphasers, it's *critical* that this behavior be avoided, or adaptation will not occur. Here's a cheat sheet with some ideas for getting past that "sleep inertia". You can carry this list, hang it up, etc., but I've always liked the idea of laying it over your face while you sleep! ☺

☼ Upon Waking

- ☐ JUMP UP!
- ☐ SING!
- ☐ CALL someone
- ☐ Do some EXERCISING
- ☐ Change CLOTHES
- ☐ WALK somewhere
- ☐ LEAVE the room immediately
- ☐ TURN ON some music, TV, or other noise
- ☐ DANCE
- ☐ Make some FOOD
- ☐ SHOWER
- ☐ Or follow your own ROUTINE:

- ☐ _____
- ☐ _____
- ☐ _____
- ☐ _____
- ☐ _____

Before you Go To Sleep

Of course, many good wake-up plans begin with taking certain actions before you go to sleep. Many of these were discussed elsewhere in this book, but here's a quick-reference list (and space to write your own ideas) of things that can be helpful to do right before you take a nap that you suspect you'll have difficulty waking up from:

🕐 Before Sleeping

- ☐ Start making some FOOD to eat when you get up
- ☐ Start an interesting PROJECT
- ☐ Do a PEP TALK
- ☐ Make PLANS with someone, in real life or online
- ☐ Or follow your own ROUTINE:

- ☐ Rotate ALARMS
- ☐ Watch the first bit of a MOVIE
- ☐ Make the room a little COLD
- ☐ Set something that needs to STAY FROZEN out

- ☐ _____
- ☐ _____
- ☐ _____
- ☐ _____
- ☐ _____

- ☐ _____
- ☐ _____
- ☐ _____
- ☐ _____
- ☐ _____

When you Get Tired

Aye, there's the rub: When you get really tired, it's hard to make decisions, especially good ones. The body tends to take the route of least resistance, which almost always means making an excuse why you should go ahead and go to sleep for a while. But the body is an opportunistic liar when it's tired; that "few minutes" or "just closing your eyes" will turn into hours before you know it, and all the hard work you've put into adapting to a polyphasic schedule so far will be for naught. The only real way to succeed in adopting a new habit as fundamental as a sleep schedule is to *give no quarter* (nor even a dime). Don't be fooled into thinking that it's okay to just rest for a second, to just lay your head down, to just sit in bed and read... like a sleazy first date, the brain/body will pull all kinds of stunts to get you into a compromising position. Of course, the best defense is still a good offense: If your "Big Fat List of Things To Do" is nice and beefy, if you can manage to have something else going on almost all the time, you'll be relatively immune from the really tricksy nudges to sleep—or to say it another way, **the human mind is a formidable adversary, but thankfully it's easily distracted**. On the other hand, even the Biggest, Fattest List can't possibly cover every second. You'll eventually hit a moment when your head is buzzing from tiredness and you realize that you're out of [suitable] things to do—what now?

The answer, of course, is another list: An Emergency Backup Big Fat List, if you will. For me, this was a section at the top of my usual Big Fat List, which I highlighted and told myself, "No matter how tired I get, I'm not allowed to even contemplate resting until I've done all these things." That's one approach. Another approach is to go through the items one at a time or pick one, but beware thinking too hard about it, since the brain's default answer will almost certainly be "Yeah, none of that looks good... let's go to sleep". **This Backup list is more of an Emergency list than a usual one; it assumes that you're tired, and that you've done or run out of all the other ideas, and that you're down to taking desperate measures**. Thus, there are some things here that are different from the other lists in this book, and which you may not want to do under normal circumstances.

You'll notice that some things which are present on most other lists are not present here—things like exercise. That's because this list assumes that you're already tired, and so it's avoiding items that might make you more tired[104]. It also avoids things that take sharp concentration, too much balance or coordination, and contact with other people—again, all assuming that you're sleep-deprived enough by the point at which you need this list that none of these is a good idea. Keep those restraints in mind as you add to or modify this list for your own needs.

There's also some rather weird items on here: for instance, there's "Talk to yourself", and "Do the Shuffle". What I mean by the former is, simply, hold a running dialog. It doesn't matter about what; just keep talking. Silence encourages sleep, whereas talking tells your brain that there's activity going on. Talking to the television, or a plant or dog or wall, works fine too. (Now that there are so many video-chat-with-people options on the Internet, I suspect those are a fantastic option as well, especially if you can talk to people whom you don't care what they think of you tomorrow!)

"The Shuffle" is an idea that was given to me by a woman I had the good fortune to talk with for a while, who did the Uberman schedule for over a year (at least; she stopped hanging out online while she was still doing it, so I don't know her end date, if indeed she's hit it yet). Due to her work, she had to drive *during* her Uberman adaptation—yeah, the mere idea gives me the shudders. But she figured out how to stave off the sleepies in a clever and amazingly effective way: By systematically tightening the muscles in the body, on rotation. Toes, feet, legs, butt, stomach, shoulders, arms, neck, fingers, toes, feet...and so forth. I'm amazed at how well this works as a short-short term, immediate solution, and I successfully used it myself when I had to drive a few times during my first Everyman adaptation and felt myself starting to fuzz out. Thanks, Heidi!

Then there's, um, "that thing grownups do". By which I mean autoerotic stimulation, or pornography, or however you like to put/have it. (I didn't put it that way on the list, because someone else might see your list, and that could be awkward.) Giggle-fits aside, the sleep portion of the brain is powerful, so it makes sense to

---

104   Exercising might be fine, as long as you don't have long to go before your next nap. But you wouldn't want to finish a round of push-ups and then realize that you're now tired *and* physically exhausted, and you've still got an hour to go!

battle it with other powerful parts of the brain, right? And we all know that the brain leaps to attention whenever there's sex involved. Before beginning any such activity, though, it's a good idea to have in mind something else to do afterwards, because you may be inclined to want to drift off in a nice relaxed haze. Still, "I'm going to organize my socks" is not nearly as compelling a personal mandate as "I'm going to thoroughly enjoy myself for ten minutes and then organize my socks." Also, keep in mind, if you plan to have an orgasm, whether orgasm typically makes you tired or gives you energy—it's different for different people! If it makes you tired, this can still be a cheap, useful way to stave of sleep for five or ten more minutes before your next scheduled nap; and if it gives you energy, well, that's just all kinds of handy then, isn't it?

For the Second Edition, I've added "Silly walks" to the list, having since discovered that inventing and practicing silly types of walking is a super-handy last-ditch sleep-dep-fender-offer. (::bows formal apology to the grammar gods::) I got this idea from my martial arts training, where stance-work exercises consisting of very specific types of stepping are practiced over and over; and I found that this is one of the things I can easily and pretty happily do for quite a long time when I'm tired. (I tried it out during one of my short re-adaptation-to-Everyman periods.) Counting steps, making geometric shapes, following or avoiding cracks or colored bits on the floor, and whatever else you can think of would probably work as well—novelty is good, and this is at base a very simple way to combine novelty, physical activity and mental distraction into an activity most of us can do even when severely impaired (walking). Credit is due, of course, to Monty Python, and the uninitiated are encouraged to look there for several iconic examples of the art of silly walking.

As you've probably noticed, there are several versions of "lists of things to do when you get tired" in this book. In my opinion, you can't have too many ideas at hand for this situation; mix them up, keep them around, and display them in whatever way works for you!

★ An Emergency Backup BFL

- ☐ Walk in CIRCLES
- ☐ Do the SHUFFLE
- ☐ Do THAT THING grownups do
- ☐ Do something MYSTERIOUS or SCARY
- ☐ SILLY WALKS
- ☐ Add your own ideas:

- ☐ Talk to YOURSELF
- ☐ SING or RECITE poetry
- ☐ Chew or suck on ICE
- ☐ Tend to PLANTS
- ☐ DUST every corner of a room

- ☐ _____
- ☐ _____
- ☐ _____
- ☐ _____
- ☐ _____

Tracking Habits and Successes

It can be hard for many people to keep track of what they've tried and what's been successful, especially when tweaking a schedule or troubleshooting a problem nap. This last Cheat Sheet is just a place for you to write things that you've tried and how often they worked, so that you can have a place to look and see that, for instance, sleeping on the couch isn't working for you, but eating lunch early is helping. In my experience, five or six times usually tells when a fix is likely to work, though don't forget that it will take a month to truly get used to any changes you make. You may also try different things to fix one certain issue, in which case just leave the extraneous "Issue" lines blank, or use them for notes.

This is also good information with which to develop a spreadsheet—if you're usually online, a Google doc or Evernote is an awesome way to track this type of data.

And you can, of course, expand this with more information—dates and times, or more singular details applicable to the type of fix you're implementing (type of food, type of alarm, etc.)—if that helps you. It depends entirely on how useful/important data gathering is to you, and how likely you are to benefit from the data later on.

Issue / Fix Needed: _____

Change made: _____

Effect of 1st try: pos / neut / neg

Effect of 2nd try: pos / neut / neg

Effect of 3rd try: pos / neut / neg

Effect of 4th try: pos / neut / neg

Effect of 5th try: pos / neut / neg

Effect of 6th try: pos / neut / neg

Issue / Fix Needed: _____

Change made: _____

Effect of 1st try: pos / neut / neg

Effect of 2nd try: pos / neut / neg

Effect of 3rd try: pos / neut / neg

Effect of 4th try: pos / neut / neg

Effect of 5th try: pos / neut / neg

Effect of 6th try: pos / neut / neg

XII. Changelog

The following changes were made for the Second Edition, in addition to the picky little tweaks that people like me can't help but make when they re-read things:

- Addition of Second Edition Introduction

- Lots of language edits to Philosophy section

- Cosmetic language and grammatical edits throughout[107];

- Correction of some minor math stuff I got wrong the first time;

- Addition of sections on "Dry or Sore Eyes", "Sore Muscles / Body Aches", "Exercise & Athletic Lifestyle", "Sleeping in Public", "Permanent Adaptation", "Readjusting to Monophasic Sleep", and the Research section devoted to Dr. Claudio Stampi

- Added definitions of "Circadian" and "Ultradian" rhythms

- Added information on the "Tesla" and other newer sleep-schedules

- Re-organized and expanded "Scheduling" section

- Expanded the section on the "Big Fat List of things to do"

- Expanded and re-organized sections on "Sleep deprivation" and "Adaptation"

- Corrected and updated the section on "Crash days"

---

107 The assistance of First Addition readers and my own grammatical OCD were both much appreciated!

- Additions to "Weight Gain and Loss" section

- Split "Re-Adjusting" into two sections on "Re-adjusting" and "Missing Sleep", to cover different types of polyphasic schedule recovery

- Redid "About the Author", because I could

- Updated Cheat Sheets

- Reformatting & design updates throughout, plus an awesome new cover

End

About the Type

This book was set in *Tisa*, a typeface created by Mitja Miklavcic in 2006. It is based on nineteenth-century slab serif wood type; a large x-height and pronounced serifs are intended to make it highly legible in both print and digital mediums.

https://www.fontfont.com/fonts/tisa

Cover text and refrences and cheat sheets are set in *Helvetica*, a typeface created in 1957 by Max Miedinger and Eduard Hoffmann. Originally called *Neue Haas Grotesk*, it was designed as neutral typeface intended to have great clarity and no tonal or stylistic meaning to its overall form.

http://www.linotype.com/526/Helvetica-family.html

Digbats/Icons were set in *Ligature Symbols*, a typeface created by Kazuyuki Motoyama in 2012. It uses semantic ligatures to insert symbols in place of typed text.

http://kudakurage.com/ligature_symbols/

Made in the USA
San Bernardino, CA
09 March 2018